Guidance and Counselling of HIV/AIDS

Guidance and Counselling of HIV/AIDS

V. Ramamurthy

AUTHORSPRESS

Worldwide Circulation through Authorspress Global Network
First Published 2004
by Authorspress

E-35/103, Jawahar Park
Laxmi Nagar, Delhi-110 092

e-mail: authorspress@yahoo.com

Typeset in NewCenturySchlbk by Chitra Computers

Guidance and Counselling of HIV/AIDS
ISBN 81-7273-184-1

Printed in India at Tarun Offset, Delhi.

Preface

HIV/AIDS is an unprecedented epidemic and public health emergency. According to recent estimates, around the world, over 33 million people are infected with HIV, and over 16 million have died of AIDS-related illnesses. In many resource-poor countries AIDS-related morbidity and mortality are causing major reversals in development, childhood mortality, and survival and life expectancy. Denial, stigma, discrimination and secrecy regarding HIV/AIDS continue to exist even though prevalence of HIV, and deaths from AIDS, are very high in many places.

It is estimated that up to 90 per cent of HIV-positive people in low-income countries do not know their HIV status. In large part, this is due to the fact that there are few voluntary counselling and testing facilities available to the populations most affected by HIV/AIDS. Realising the fact, nowadays, governments, international agencies, and non-governmental organisations are incorporating HIV testing and counselling programme on a broader and radically larger scale in their HIV/AIDS interventions, in order to meet an increasing global demand for access to care and prevention services.

HIV counselling has been proved effective in various ways. It empowers individuals to prevent transmission of HIV by enabling them to cope with the personal implications of an HIV diagnosis and to make informed personal decisions, including those related to sexuality and reproduction. It provides psycho-social and spiritual support to those who are affected and should assist clients to make decisions that will improve the quality of their lives. It can help the affected persons adopt new lifestyles, and assist them to retain their identities, independence, privacy, social status and self-worth. This can then reduce the risk of negative outcomes, re-infection, and transmission of infection to others.

The development of HIV counselling services in response to an ever increasing demand for them requires sustained counselling training programmes and curricula that are consistent with the emerging needs of the HIV affected community. As there is a tendency to be flooded with diverse counselling approaches and techniques derived from different scientific fields, the focus of counselling training should be on the basic skills and techniques.

The present volume provides a comprehensive analysis of HIV counselling practices available today. It contains information, ideas and suggestions for those who work with HIV clients and who want to improve their knowledge and skills in counselling in STD/HIV prevention, safer sex, pre- and post-HIV antibody testing and other issues related to the subject. It highlights the importance of ethical, innovative and pragmatic approaches to increase access to and uptake of HIV counselling services and thereby to enhance efforts to promote HIV prevention, care and treatment.

The book is designed to help counsellors, health workers, educators and all those working in STD/HIV/AIDS, to improve the effectiveness of their work and the quality of lives of the people they aim to support.

Editor

Contents

	Preface	*v*
1.	HIV/AIDS: Discrimination and Denial	1
2.	Awareness Strategies	23
3.	Guidance and Counselling of HIV/AIDS	69
4.	Ethical Partner Counselling	133
5.	Infant Feeding	193
6.	Survival Guidance for HIV Patients	215
7.	Monitoring HIV/AIDS Care	249
	Bibliography	279
	Index	285

1

HIV/AIDS: Discrimination and Denial

Acquired Immune Deficiency Syndrome (AIDS) is caused by Human Immuno-deficiency Virus (HIV), a virus which kills or impairs cells in the immune system, destroying the body's ability to fight infections and cancers. The virus is transmitted horizontally and vertically. "Horizontal" transmission occurs during heterosexual intercourse and between men who have sex with men (MSM) when no barrier method (i.e., condom) is used during intercourse with an HIV-infected person. It is also transmitted between injecting drug users (IDU) from sharing infected needles. "Vertical" transmission occurs between mothers and their children during or after pregnancy. Approximately one in three children (0-2 years) will contract HIV from infected mothers. The most typical mode of transmission varies within regions and countries but the regional trends do highlight something of the scale of the problem.

The first cases of AIDS are believed to date as far back as the 1930's but only in the 1980's did it reach global proportions. According to recent estimates about 34.3 million people around the world are living with HIV/AIDS and over 5 million people are newly infected each year and more than 6 thousand lives are lost every day to the disease; 3. 8 million children (aged 0-14) have died since 1980 and nearly 13 million children have been orphaned as a result of the epidemic. The horrifying situation is most starkly apparent in Sub Sahara Africa (SSA), which accounts for over 70 per cent of people infected globally. Whilst strategies to combat HIV/AIDS are improving and recent medical advancements in prevention and care have been considerable, there is a long way to go to limit further spread of the disease and help those most crippled by the epidemic.

AIDS infects people irrespective of economic background but the epidemic is most keenly felt by those with the least resources to tackle it. One-third of the world's population lacks access to basic medication, let alone the specialised treatments required for HIV/AIDS. Something little short of miracle is required to cope with the enormous battle ahead, and for SSA in particular only a concerted international effort is going to have any kind of impact.

HIV/AIDS has severely undermined the development of many countries, in terms of individual suffering and loss, as well as knock-on effects to families, communities, economies, medical services, businesses, public services and society as a whole. At the macroeconomic level, the epidemic has impacted national economic growth in a number of countries, e.g., Tanzania has experienced a 15 to 25 per cent fall in GDP as a result of the AIDS epidemic. This is due to a number of reasons.

The epidemic absorbs a lot of funds for the provision of basic health care and prevention services, e.g., in Rwanda in 1995 an estimated 66 per cent of public health expenditure was for HIV/ AIDS patients. Increasingly stretched resources mean that the provision of health care for other patients is also severely reduced. Government revenues and private savings are reduced by these health costs, as well as due to the costs of implementing related regulatory and social security systems. Such costs slow investment in employment creation and capital intensive sectors.

The impacts on the workplace are also considerable. For example, AIDS-related increases in mortality are predicted to reduce workforces globally by 11.5 million people by the year 2020 and some African work forces will fall by as much as 20 per cent of existing levels. Human resources, especially in key sectors such as teaching and health care, are cut back and rural areas are particularly effected as people are less willing to work in areas with poor access to services.

The quantity and quality of labour has declined for a number of reasons, such as AIDS related increases in absenteeism and mortality, as well as from reduced capacity in education and health care, and human resources training. Certain sectors are more effected than others, e.g., transport, fishing, mining, tourism, agriculture and construction. This is because the work is typically seasonal or involves considerable travel away from home and families, factors associated with higher levels of risky behaviour in individuals.

The epidemic is having a devastating effect on agricultural output, e.g., Zimbabwe's maize production has dropped by 61 per cent because of AIDS-related losses in staff. Agriculture is the largest industry in Africa and an important form of subsistence for many developing countries, yet farmers are being forced to switch to less labour intensive crops, which directly impacts on the security of food supply.

Military/civilian interaction is also instrumental in spreading HIV/AIDS. Armed forces are highly mobile, and soldiers are known to solicit commercial sex, as well as use rape as a weapon of war. Refugee populations are especially vulnerable to such activities. The risk of HIV infection is estimated at six times higher in refugee camps than outside. As a result of their close involvement with infected individuals in areas of conflict peace-keeping forces are also at risk of infection.

Several African countries currently face armed conflict, food emergencies, inadequate water supply and sanitation, droughts and floods. HIV/AIDS severely exacerbates the political instability and insecurity in SSA. In 1999, 2 million people were killed by HIV/AIDS in SSA as compared to the 200.000 thousand who die each year from armed conflict.

At the microeconomic and local level, earnings, savings and disposable income are likely to fall with greater numbers of people facing the financial burden associated to HIV/AIDS care and treatment. Young adults (15-49), especially women, display high rates of infection, from Sexually Transmitted Diseases (STDs) as well as HIV. They often lack the knowledge and resources to protect themselves and others. In the past, the highest number of infected cases were found in men, however, women are showing increased levels of infection.

In 1999, women accounted for 49 per cent of new infections and more than 50 per cent of AIDS related deaths. Of the cumulative total of adult deaths (18.8 million) since the beginning of the pandemic more than 51 per cent were women. The infection impacts on women's health, physical and mental well-being, raises the risk of mother to child transmission, affects their ability to be mothers and careers, and limits their educational and employment opportunities. Children also face infection, being orphaned, and suffer untold psychological effects because of the abuse, alienation, stigma and discrimination which is frequently borne by individuals associated with the disease. Such pressures mean that children tend to drop out early from school, forcing them to become providers for themselves and their families. Reduced access to education and loss of teachers has a direct impact upon the skills and learning of young people, further diminishing their ability to develop as "healthy" members of society.

The family structure is effected as the need for extended families to support infected individuals and orphaned children is enhanced. However, these traditional structures are weakening in many developing and transitional countries due to urbanisation and migratory changes. The elderly are also likely to bear an increasing burden as a result, e.g., care of infected people, orphaned children, and remaining in the work-place for longer period. Marginalised people e.g. the poor, minorities, migrants, indigenous people, IDUs, sex workers, people with disabilities, MSM, prisoners, all have to cope with an increasing incidence of HIV/AIDS. Limited economic, political and social influence, as well as lack of access to basic services reduces an individual's ability to combat the disease.

HIV/AIDS is a threat to the growth of the community. As the epidemic spreads, every affected country loses its most productive, vibrant citizens. Not only do families lose parents, spouses and breadwinners, societies lose their farmers, teachers, health-care workers, managers, spiritual leaders, members of religious organisations and others who make the community strong.

HIV/AIDS is a threat to efforts to fight poverty. As increasing numbers of the sick and dying need health and hospital care, and as more families lose time and money through sickness or caregiving responsibilities, already meagre family, community and national budgets are drying up.

HIV/AIDS is a threat to human dignity. As heads of households lose their ability to provide, lose their social standing, suffer the indignities of debilitating illnesses and see their families fall further into poverty, many lose all hope. Where stigma and discrimination prevail, people with HIV and AIDS are shunned, filled with guilt and often deny the truth, even at the risk of spreading HIV to others. Children and wives who experience the illness or death of loved ones, and who must suddenly fend for themselves, are often subjected to abandonment, abuse and exploitation.

HIV/AIDS is a threat to family life and spiritual well-being. As young men and women fall ill and die, they often suffer spiritual anguish, social isolation and physical and economic hardship. They also leave behind grieving children, spouses and friends who call out for comfort and practical guidance.

HIV-RELATED STIGMA AND DISCRIMINATION

Jonathan Mann, the former director of the WHO Global Programme on AIDS, identified three phases of the HIV/AIDS epidemic: the epidemic of HIV, the epidemic of AIDS, and the epidemic of stigma, discrimination, and denial. According to him third phase is "as central to the global AIDS challenge as the disease itself".

Despite international efforts to tackle HIV/AIDS, stigma and discrimination (S&D) remain among the most poorly understood aspects of the epidemic—stigma as a "continuing challenge" that prevents concerted action at community, national, and global levels. This poor understanding is due in part to the complexity and diversity of S&D, but also in part to limitations in current thinking within the field and the inadequacy of available theoretical and methodological tools.

To understand the ways in which HIV/AIDS-related S&D appear and the contexts in which they occur, we first need to understand how they interact with pre-existing S&D associated with sexuality, gender, race, and poverty. HIV/AIDS-related S&D also interact with pre-existing fears about contagion and disease. Early AIDS metaphors—as death, as horror, as punishment, as guilt, as shame, as otherness—have exacerbated these fears, reinforcing and legitimising stigmatisation and discrimination.

Sex-related Stigma

HIV/AIDS-related S&D are most closely related to sexual stigma. This is because HIV is mainly sexually transmitted and in most areas of the world, the epidemic initially affected populations whose sexual practices or identities are different from the "norm." HIV/AIDS-related S&D has therefore appropriated and reinforced pre-existing sexual stigma associated with sexually transmitted diseases, homosexuality, promiscuity, prostitution, and sexual "deviance".

The belief that homosexuals are to blame for the epidemic or that homosexuals are the only group at risk of HIV is still common. Promiscuous sexual behaviour by women is also commonly believed to be responsible for the heterosexual epidemic, regardless of the epidemiological reality. In Brazil, for example, where surveillance data have shown high rates of HIV infection among monogamous married women, HIV-positive women are still widely perceived to be sexually promiscuous.

Gender-related Stigma

HIV/AIDS-related S&D are also linked to gender-related stigma. The impact of HIV/AIDS-related S&D on women reinforces pre-existing economic, educational, cultural, and social disadvantages and unequal access to information and services. In settings where heterosexual transmission is significant, the spread of HIV infection has been associated with female sexual behaviour that is not consistent with gender norms. For example, prostitution is widely perceived as non-normative female behaviour, and female sex workers are often identified as "vectors" of infection who put at risk their clients and their clients' sexual partners. Equally, in many settings, men are blamed for heterosexual transmission, because of assumptions about male sexual behaviour, such as men's preference or need for multiple sexual partners.

Race-related Stigma

Racial and ethnic S&D also interact with HIV/AIDS-related S&D, and the epidemic has been characterised both by racist assumptions about "African sexuality" and by perceptions in the developing world of the West's "immoral behaviour." Racial and ethnic S&D contribute to the marginalisation of minority population groups, increasing their vulnerability to HIV/AIDS, which in turn exacerbates stigmatisation and discrimination.

Class-related Stigma

The HIV/AIDS epidemic has developed during a period of rapid globalisation and growing polarisation between the rich and the poor. New forms of social exclusion associated with these global changes have reinforced pre-existing social inequalities and stigmatisation of the poor, homeless, landless, and jobless. As a result, poverty increases vulnerability to HIV/AIDS, and HIV/AIDS exacerbates poverty. HIV/AIDS-related S&D interacts with pre-existing S&D associated with economic marginalisation. In some contexts, the epidemic has been characterised by assumptions about the rich, and HIV/AIDS has been associated with affluent lifestyles.

Fear-related Stigma

HIV/AIDS is a life-threatening illness that people are afraid of contracting. The various metaphors associated with AIDS have also contributed to the perception of HIV/AIDS as a disease that affects "others," especially those who are already stigmatised because of their sexual behaviour, gender, race, or socio-economic status, and have enabled some people to deny that they personally could be at risk or affected. HIV/AIDS-related S&D is, therefore, the result of interaction between diverse pre-existing sources of S&D and fear of contagion and disease. The pre-existing sources, such as those related to gender, sexuality, and class, often overlap and reinforce one another. This interaction has contributed to the deep-rooted nature of HIV/AIDS-related S&D, limiting our ability to develop effective responses. It has also created a vicious circle of S&D, which works in two ways.

First, because HIV/AIDS is associated with marginalised behaviours and groups, all individuals with HIV/AIDS are assumed to be from marginalised groups and some may be stigmatised in a way that they were not before. For example, in some settings, men may fear revealing their HIV status because it will be assumed that they are homosexual. Similarly, women may fear revealing their zero-status because they may be labelled as "promiscuous" or sex workers and stigmatised as such.

Second, HIV/AIDS exacerbates the stigmatisation of individuals and groups who are already oppressed and marginalised, which increases their vulnerability to HIV/AIDS, and which in turn causes them to be further stigmatised and marginalised.

Manifestations of Stigma and Discrimination

HIV/AIDS-related S&D take different forms and are manifested at different levels—societal, community and individual—and in different contexts.

Legal levels

HIV/AIDS-related S&D in society is commonly manifested in the form of laws, policies, and administrative procedures, which are often justified as necessary to protect the "general population". Examples of stigmatising and discriminatory measures include compulsory screening and testing, compulsory notification of AIDS cases, restrictions of the right to anonymity, prohibition of PLHA from certain occupations, and medical examination, isolation, detention and compulsory treatment of infected persons.

One important example concerns limitations on international travel and migration. Despite widespread agreement that laws to prevent freedom of movement of people living with HIV/AIDS (PLHA) are ineffective public health measures, many countries have adopted policies restricting travel and migration.

Discriminatory practices include mandatory HIV testing for individuals seeking work permits, the requirement that individuals seeking tourist visas declare their HIV serostatus, and denial of entry to PLHA carrying medical drugs for HIV/AIDS treatment. Foreigners have been deported from a diverse range of countries after the authorities have discovered that they are HIV-positive.

HIV/AIDS-related S&D reinforces existing prejudice toward foreigners or marginalised groups. For example, travellers from countries worst affected by the epidemic, or whose appearance makes others think they are gay men or sex workers, may be subject to additional questioning and physical searches. Foreign nationals engaged in sex work may be deported because of the risk they are said to pose to local clients. Early on in the epidemic, there were many reports of African students in Europe and Asia being detained or deported in this way.

Some governments, recognising that such measures are ineffective, have introduced legislation to protect the rights of PLHA to education, employment, confidentiality, information, and treatment. However, even when supportive legislation exists, it is not always enforced. The failure of governments to protect the rights of PLHA through legislation or to enforce existing legislation has been described as a form of discrimination by neglect, as has the failure to provide effective prevention, treatment and care for those most vulnerable to HIV/AIDS and for PLHA.

Institutional levels

Education and schools: Children with HIV/AIDS or associated with HIV through infected family members have been stigmatised and discriminated against in educational settings in many countries. Stigma has led to teasing by classmates of HIV-positive school children or children associated with HIV. Discrimination against HIV-positive children in the USA and Brazil, including exclusion from collective activities or expulsion from school, has led to non-discrimination legislation.

However, less concern has been shown for young people who are perceived to be responsible for their HIV infection and who are already stigmatised and discriminated against because they are sexually active, homosexual, or drug users. In the USA, for example, HIV-positive young gay men have been expelled from school and, in some cases, subjected to violence.

Employment and the workplace: Such discriminatory practices as pre-employment screening, denial of employment to individuals who test positive, termination of employment of PLHA, and stigmatisation of PLHA who are open about their serostatus have been reported from developed and developing countries. There have been reports of workers refusing to work next to those with HIV or AIDS or those perceived to be PLHA.

Schemes providing medical assistance and pensions to employees have come under increasing pressure in countries seriously affected by HIV/AIDS, and some companies have used this as a reason to deny employment to PLHA. Few companies have developed strategies to combat S&D or defined their responsibilities toward employees with HIV.

Health care systems: There have been many reports from health care settings of HIV testing without consent, breaches of confidentiality, and denial of treatment and care. Failure to respect confidentiality by clearly identifying patients with HIV/AIDS, revealing serostatus to relatives without prior consent, or releasing information to the media or police appear to be problems in some health service. Factors contributing to these stigmatising and discriminatory responses include lack of knowledge, moral attitudes, and perceptions that caring for PLHA is pointless because HIV/AIDS is incurable.

HIV/AIDS programmes: HIV/AIDS policies and programmes may inadvertently contribute to stigmatisation and discrimination by differentiating between the "general population" and "high-risk populations," prioritising actions to prevent HIV spreading to the former from the latter. This approach is often justified in terms of avoiding stigmatisation of "high-risk populations," since targeting such populations is believed to reinforce the association of HIV/AIDS with marginalised groups.

However, focusing on programmes for the "general population" may also reinforce the perception that it is less important to protect populations that practice "high-risk" behaviours than the "innocent and unsuspecting" general population. It may also result in discrimination against marginalised groups, since those at greatest risk do not receive the resources they need.

Furthermore, in some settings, allocating resources on the basis of acceptability rather than of need may be a deliberate policy, because of racism, homophobia, or negative attitudes toward marginalised groups. For example, government expenditure in most Latin American countries does not reflect the fact that HIV/AIDS has a disproportionate impact on homosexually and bisexually active men in these countries.

Religious institutions: In some contexts, HIV/AIDS-related S&D has been reinforced by religious leaders and organisations, which have used their power to maintain the *status quo* rather than to challenge negative attitudes toward marginalised groups and PLHA. For example, at the international symposium Religious Health Organisations Break the Silence on HIV/AIDS, organised by the African Regional Forum of Religious Health Organisations during the 13th International AIDS Conference in July 2000, it was noted that religious doctrines, moral and ethical positions regarding sexual behaviour, sexism and homophobia, and denial of the realities of HIV/AIDS have helped create the perception that those infected have sinned and deserve their "punishment," increasing the stigma associated with HIV/AIDS.

Community levels

In societies with cultural systems that place greater emphasis on individualism, HIV/AIDS may be perceived as the result of personal irresponsibility, and thus individuals are blamed for contracting the infection. In contrast, in societies where cultural systems place greater emphasis on collectivism, HIV/AIDS may be perceived as bringing shame on the family and community.

The type of cultural system and where it fits along the continuum of individualism and collectivism will therefore influence the ways in which communities respond to HIV/AIDS and the ways in which S&D are manifested. Local cultural beliefs and explanations about disease and the causes of disease may also contribute to HIV/AIDS-related S&D. For example, where illness is believed to be the result of "immoral" or "improper" behaviour, HIV/AIDS may reinforce pre-existing stigma of those whose behaviour is considered to be "deviant".

HIV/AIDS-related S&D in families and communities is commonly manifested in the form of blame, scape goating, and punishment. Communities often shun or gossip about those perceived to have HIV or AIDS. In more extreme cases, it has taken the form of violence. For example, there have been reports from many countries of attacks on men who are assumed to be gay, of violence toward sex workers and street children in Brazil and of HIV/AIDS-related murders in Colombia, India, Ethiopia, South Africa, and Thailand.

Family levels

The family is the main source of care and support for PLHA in most developing countries. However, negative family responses are common. Infected individuals often experience S&D in the home, and women are often more likely to be badly treated than men or children. Negative community and family responses to women with HIV/AIDS include blame, rejection, and loss of children and home.

Since HIV/AIDS-related S&D reinforce and interact with pre-existing S&D, families may reject PLHA not only because of their HIV status but also because HIV/AIDS is associated with promiscuity, homosexuality, and drug use. In many cases, HIV/AIDS-related S&D has been extended to families, neighbours and friends of PLHA. This 'secondary' stigmatisation and discrimination has played an important role in creating and reinforcing social isolation of those affected by the epidemic, such as the children and partners of PLHA.

Individual levels

In individuals, the way in which HIV/AIDS-related S&D are manifested depends on family and social support and the degree to which people are able to be open about such issues as their sexuality as well as their serostatus. In contexts where HIV/AIDS is highly stigmatised, fear of HIV/AIDS-related S&D may cause individuals to isolate themselves to the extent that they no longer feel part of civil society and are unable to gain access the services and support they need. This has been called internalised stigma. In extreme cases, this has led to premature death through suicide.

Even when laws exist to protect PLHA rights and confidentiality, few individuals are willing to litigate for fear that this will result in disclosure of their identity and HIV status. Given widespread negative community and family responses, many people choose not to know or reveal their serostatus.

Individuals who are already marginalised may be fearful of negative or hostile reactions from others, regardless of their serostatus, reflecting the interaction between HIV/AIDS-related and pre-existing sources of S&D. Fear of telling the family about their homosexuality has been cited by HIV-positive men in Mexico and Brazil as equal to the fear of revealing their serostatus. Similar fears have been reported from a range of countries by sex workers and injecting drug users. Even when the family response is positive, fear of stigmatisation and discrimination by the community may mean that an individual's serostatus is not revealed outside the home.

Developing a New Conceptual Framework

HIV/AIDS-related S&D are linked to the actions and attitudes of families, communities, and societies. However, current thinking largely focuses on S&D as individual processes—or as what some individuals do to other individuals—rather than as social processes. The dominant definition describes stigma as a "discrediting attribute" and stigmatised individuals as those who possess an "undesirable difference," and ignores aspects that describe stigma as something that is socially constructed. This has resulted in the notion that stigma is a static individual feature or characteristic, limiting analysis of the underlying causes and possible responses to HIV/AIDS-related S&D. We need to move beyond current thinking toward a conceptual framework that is based on an understanding that S&D are social processes and that, consequently, S&D can be resisted and challenged by social action.

Social and political theory can help us to understand that stigmatisation and discrimination are not isolated phenomena or the expression of individual attitudes, but are social processes used to create and maintain social control and to produce and reproduce social inequality.

Stigma is something that is "produced" and used to help order society. For example, most societies achieve conformity by contrasting those who are "normal" with those who are "different" or "deviant." Cultures therefore produce "difference" in order to achieve social control. In many non-Western societies, local knowledge systems may perform the same function at a more localised level.

Similarly, concepts of symbolic violence and hegemony highlight the role of stigmatisation in establishing social order and control, and identify stigmatisation as part of the social struggle for power. Symbolic violence is a process where words, images and practices promote the interests of dominant groups, and hegemony is achieved through the use of political, social and cultural forces to promote dominant meanings and values that legitimise unequal social structures.

So all cultural meanings and practices embody interests and are used to enhance social distinctions between individuals, groups, and institutions. Sociological analyses of discrimination are also useful because they emphasise the structural aspects of discrimination and "concentrate on patterns of dominance and oppression, viewed as expressions of a struggle for power and privilege."

Following from the notion that stigmatisation is a process that involves identifying differences between groups of people, and using these differences to determine where groups fit into structures of power, is the idea that stigma and discrimination are used to produce and reproduce social inequality. Stigmatisation, therefore, not only helps to create difference but also plays a key role in transforming difference based on class, gender, race, ethnicity, or sexuality into social inequality. Stigmatisation is also used by dominant groups to legitimise and perpetuate inequalities, and concepts of symbolic violence and hegemony can also help us understand how it is that those who are stigmatised and discriminated against so often accept, and even internalise, the stigma to which they are subjected. This is because the processes of symbolic violence and hegemony convince the dominated to accept existing hierarchies and allow social hierarchies to persist over generations, without generating conscious recognition from those who are dominated.

In addition, these processes limit the ability of oppressed and stigmatised groups and individuals to resist the forces that discriminate against them.

An understanding of stigmatisation and discrimination as political and social processes can also help us to reconsider responses to HIV/AIDS-related S&D. For example, identity theory suggests that those who are stigmatised can take action to resist the forces that discriminate against them. Those who are marginalised generate "resistance identities" and use them to build a new identity that redefines their position in society and thus seeks the transformation of overall social structure. This would include resistance through mobilisation of movements, at community, national, and international levels, aimed at social change.

These ideas offer important insights for reconceptualising HIV/AIDS-related stigmatisation and discrimination within a broader social, cultural, political, and economic framework rather than as individual processes. They offer a framework for understanding S&D as social processes that are used to create a social hierarchy by differentiating between the stigmatised and the nonstigmatised, as well as to produce and reproduce social inequalities and to make these inequalities seem reasonable.

Such a framework improves our ability to analyse the causes of S&D and the ways in which HIV/AIDS S&D interact with and reinforce pre-existing S&D and social exclusion. More important, a better understanding of the processes that produce S&D, as well as of the processes that produce resistance to S&D, would enable us to develop more effective responses to HIV/AIDS-related S&D.

A new way of thinking has implications for the way in which research and interventions to address HIV/AIDS-related S&D are framed and implemented. It implies the need for a broader approach, in which existing conceptual frameworks and intervention models that focus on the individual are complemented by:

a) *New approaches to research:* ways of understanding HIV/AIDS-related S&D that take account of social, cultural, political, and economic determinants.

b) *New approaches to programming and interventions*: ways of responding to HIV/AIDS-related S&D that engage societies, communities, and those who suffer stigmatisation and discrimination.

New approaches to research

Further development of the conceptual framework encourage research in three areas: exploratory and hypothesis-generating studies to inform investigative studies, investigative studies to inform policy and strategy, and strategic and policy-oriented studies to inform programme implementation. Such research would emphasise indepth work that focuses on the social context rather than studies that examine the behavioural and psychological dimensions of HIV/AIDS-related S& D. The ultimate purpose of this research, including exploratory and investigative studies that are not directly linked to interventions, should be to support the development of policies and programmes that will reduce HIV/AIDS-related S&D.

i) *Exploratory and hypothesis-generating studies.* Research is required:

   a) To identify the environmental or structural sources of S&D and the ways in which they are manifested through case studies and qualitative community research.

   b) To identify and develop new concepts and understanding that encompass the social, cultural, political, and economic determinants and consequences of HIV/AIDS-related S&D, and that will be relevant for policies and programmes in different cultures and contexts.

   c) To review the adequacy and appropriateness of concepts and understanding over time, in the light of changing needs, priorities, and circumstances that have an impact on HIV/AIDS-related S&D.

d) To contribute to understanding of the processes of change, social movements, and cultural transformation in response to HIV and AIDS-related S&D.

ii) *Investigative studies.* Research is required:

a) To investigate social processes in a range of different contexts to enable comparisons to be made and to develop an understanding of aspects of HIV/AIDS-related S&D that are locally specific, as well as aspects that cut across cultural and national boundaries.

b) To identify opportunities and future priorities for intervention, including environmental and structural interventions.

c) To provide insights into the reasons for the successes and failures of interventions intended to reduce S&D. This requires identifying new tools for evaluating environmental and structural interventions.

d) To investigate other strategies and interventions, such as home-based care, family counselling, and availability of effective treatment, that are not primarily intended to address S&D but may do so indirectly, to assess the extent to which they contribute to reducing S&D.

iii) *Strategic and policy-oriented studies.* Research is required:

a) To identify the policy and programme elements and interventions that contribute to effective responses to HIV/AIDS-related S&D.

b) To identify how these can best be put into operation and the likely outcomes of specific approaches to programme implementation.

c) To improve understanding of how program implementation and the potential for replication and scaling up of successful approaches are influenced by the broader policy and social context.

New approaches to programming and interventions

Responding to HIV/AIDS-related S&D as manifestations of power, inequality, and exclusion implies developing environmental and structural interventions to change the context within which individuals and communities respond to HIV/AIDS, in addition to individual interventions. Individual psychological approaches alone will not achieve changes in S&D and must be complemented by action to address structural and environmental constraints.

Environmental interventions: Issues to consider include developing programmes that aim to achieve social and community change rather than just individual behaviour change, drawing on the experience of community mobilisation and social transformation in other areas. Priority should be given to approaches that aim to strengthen capacity for resistance among stigmatised and marginalised groups, since empirical evidence indicates that some of the most effective responses to the HIV/AIDS epidemic have been those where affected communities have mobilised themselves to fight stigma, discrimination, and oppression.

Particular attention should be paid to learning lessons from the experience of community organisation and of empowering or "unleashing the power of resistance" of stigmatised populations and communities. Examples relevant to HIV/AIDS include the Greater Involvement of People Living with or Affected by HIV/AIDS (GIPA) principle, which promotes the active involvement of PLHA in government ministries and civil society organisations to both empower PLHA and to encourage positive perceptions of PLHA, and support for PLHA organisations and networks, which have enabled people living with HIV/AIDS to demand recognition of their existence, needs, and rights.

Organising has also enabled those who are marginalised to challenge discrimination and to lobby for changes in laws and policies. For example, sex worker unions have challenged police persecution, gay men's organisations have played a significant role in advocating for access to treatment, and women's organisations have lobbied for changes in the inheritance rights of widows. Such activities, designed to empower marginalised groups, should complement ongoing efforts to change individual attitudes toward PLHA and those affected by the epidemic through, for example, media campaigns promoting tolerance and compassion.

Useful lessons could be learned from efforts to address S&D associated with other issues, such as mental health and leprosy. In Scotland, for example, providing the community with information and encouraging greater day-to-day contact with people with mental illness helped to reduce stigmatisation of mental illness, and a national campaign in the UK to educate the public about mental illness resulted in more positive attitudes and greater willingness to seek treatment from health professionals. In Tanzania, a health education campaign designed to reduce the stigma of leprosy improved community attitudes in terms of, for example, greater willingness to share food or shake hands with a person with leprosy. Finally, there is a need to develop advocacy models to address HIV/AIDS-related S&D, drawing on the experience of community mobilisation, empowerment, and social transformation.

Structural interventions: Priority should be given to developing a legal and policy framework that protects the human rights of PLHA and those affected by the epidemic and that helps to mitigate the impact of HIV/AIDS-related S&D. Useful lessons about structural interventions are available from countries that have implemented protective legal and policy frameworks, such as the 100 per cent condom programmes in Thailand, Cambodia, and the Dominican Republic, where the government introduced policies requiring bar owners to promote condom use by clients of sex workers. This approach appears to have changed social norms toward unprotected sex with sex workers and, more important, provided structural protection to enable sex workers to negotiate condom use.

REFERENCES

Aggleton, P. and I. Warwick, 1999, *Household and Community Responses to HIV and AIDS in Developing Countries: Findings from Multi-site Studies*, Geneva, UNAIDS.

Altman, D., *Power and Community: Organisational and Cultural Responses to AIDS*, London: Taylor and Francis, 1994.

Bharat, S. and P. Aggleton, "Facing the challenge: Household responses to AIDS in India," *AIDS Care* 11:33-46, 1999.

Blendon, R.J. and K. Donelan. 1988. "Discrimination against people with AIDS," *American Journal of Public Health* 319:1022-1026.

Bourdieu, P. and J-C. Passeron. 1977. *Reproduction in Education, Society and Culture*, London: Sage.

Castells, M., *The Network Society*, Oxford: Blackwell Publishers, Inc., 1996.

Corbett, E.L., Watt, C.J., Walker, N., etal., "The growing burden of tuberculosis: global trends and interactions with the HIV epidemic", *Archives of Internal Medicine*, 163:100-921, 2003.

Gagnon, J.H. and W. Simon, *Sexual Conduct*, Chicago: Aldine, 1973.

Gilmore, N. and M.A. Somerville, "Stigmatisation, scapegoating and discrimination in sexually transmitted diseases, overcoming 'them' and 'us'," *Social Science and Medicine*, 39:1339-1358, 1994.

Gostin, L.O. and Z. Lazzarini, *Human Rights and Public Health in the AIDS Pandemic*, New York: Oxford University Press, 1997.

ILO, *Action Against HIV/AIDS A Draft Framework for Global and Regional initiatives*, International Labour Organisation. Geneva, November 1999.

Kegeles, S.M. etal., "Perceptions of AIDS, the continuing saga of AIDS-related stigma," *AIDS* 3(suppl.1):S253-S258, 1989.

Kirp, D.L. and R. Bayer (ed.), 1992, *AIDS in the Industrialised Democracies*, New Brunswick, NJ: Rutgers University Press.

Malcolm, A. et al., "HIV and AIDS-related stigmatisation and discrimination: its form and contexts," *Critical Public Health* 8(4):347-370, 1998.

Mann, J., D.J.M. Tarantola, and T.W. Netter (ed.), *AIDS in the World*, Boston, MA: Harvard University Press, 1992.

Mujeeb, S. 1999. "Human right violations of PLWA/HIV by their family members," posting to *SEA-AIDS*, Tue, 06 Jul 1999.

Parker, R.,"Administering the epidemic: HIV/AIDS policy, models of development and international health in the late-twentieth century," in *Globalisation, Health and Identity: The Fallacy of the Level Playing Field*, ed. L.M. Whiteford and L. Manderson. Boulder, CO: Lynne Rienner Publishing, pp. 39-55, 2000.

______________ , Aggleton, P., etal, *HIV/AIDS-related Stigma and Discrimination: A Conceptual Framework and an Agenda for Action*, The Population Council Inc., 2002.

Sweat, M. and J. Dennison, "Reducing HIV incidence in developing countries with structural and environmental interventions," *AIDS* 9(suppl. A): S225-257, 1995.

Tirelli, U. etal, "HIV and discrimination", *British Medical Journal* 303:582, 1991.

Tarantola, and T.W. Netter. Boston, MA: Harvard University Press. UNAIDS, *HIV and AIDS-related stigmatisation, discrimination and denial: forms, contexts and determinants*, research studies from Uganda and India (prepared for UNAIDS by Peter Aggleton), Geneva, UNAIDS, 2000.

UNAIDS, Report on the global HIV/AIDS Epidemic, June 2000.

USAID, *USAID Concept Paper: Combating HIV/AIDS Stigma, Discrimination and Denial*, 2000.

World Bank, *Confronting AIDS: Public Priorities in a Global Epidemic*, New York: Oxford University Press, 1997.

______________ , *Confronting AIDS: Public Priorities in a Global Epidemic*, A World Bank Policy Research Report, Oxford University Press, 1997.

2

Awareness Strategies

HIV/AIDS, first described 20 years ago, has devastated the world, and especially Sub-Saharan Africa, where it has had an unprecedented impact on all sectors (health, agriculture, education, defence, economy, demographics, child survival, and orphanhood). There are treatments to control opportunistic infections, ameliorate symptoms, and slow the progress of the disease, but these are not widely available or accessible. There is still no cure or vaccine, though research efforts are continuing in those areas.

REASONS FOR INCREASED SPREAD OF HIV/AIDS

The major reasons for increased infection rate of HIV/AIDS include:

i) *Poverty:* Due to economic hardships, many young women exchange sex for money and other gifts. The "sugar daddy" phenomenon is rampant, even though it is not necessarily condoned. A sugar daddy is a man who pays a girlfriend money or favors in exchange for sex and a romantic relationship. Girls who have lost their parents, and who have the responsibility of caring for their siblings, are also forced to exchange sex for money, since they have few skills through which they can earn a reasonable living. Some girls become 'professional' sex workers. They have intercourse with many different sexual partners without using any kind of protection against sexually transmitted infections (STIs) or HIV/AIDS. The high prevalence of STIs, combined with limited availability of STI services and treatment, may increase exposure to and transmission of HIV.

ii) *Culture:* In some countries, village chiefs still inherit multiple wives from previous chiefs without considering HIV testing. While polygamy is common, it was not associated with increased risk of HIV infection in our preliminary analyses. In some villages, husbands and wives swap partners on certain days, a practice that increases risk of HIV transmission and should be discouraged. Many men believe that they need frequent sex to maintain their manhood, including during the traditional period of sexual abstinence of lactating mothers, usually for about 18 months postpartum. During this time, it has been acceptable for the fathers to have sex with "free women" or prostitutes, and then return to sexual relations with their wives after weaning, a practice that can promote the spread of HIV.

iii) Gender: Women are dependent on men who take them as wives or girlfriends. They have little control over where, when, or even how to have sex. In some countries, women are not allowed to talk openly about sexual matters, and it is particularly difficult for a woman to initiate discussions about using condoms.

iv) *Lack of aiwareness*: Although much information about HIV/AIDS has been disseminated, many people still do not know or understand the facts. Confusion exists because numerous myths have circulated, such as, "HIV/AIDS is caused by having sex with relatives."

v) *Failure to change behavior*: The pleasure of sex outweighs the risk for some people, thus exposing them to danger. Many people lack self-control. Due to gender inequities in the society, women have little say in what measures are taken to make sex "safe."

vi) *Wars and political instability*: Periods of political instability in developing countries and the subsequent breakdown of societal order created situations where women and girls were raped and abused, in a context with no legal protection and little access to medical care.

vii) *Inaccessibility to Short Course Antiretroviral Drugs (ARVs) for PMTCT*: Many HIV-infected persons in developing countries do not have access to anti-retrovirals (ARVs) due to the high cost, limited availability, and the fact that ARV treatment of AIDS is lifelong. Although nevirapine (NVP) treatment for PMTCT is currently available free of charge from Axios International for developing countries, it is accessible to only a very small proportion of HIVinfected pregnant women. Since pregnant women often deliver at a different health facility from the one where they receive HIV testing as part of prenatal care, there is a great need to make PMTCT services available at all facilities.

HIV/AIDS is transmitted through the following body fluids: blood, semen, vaginal secretions, and breast milk. The following table depicts the percentage of infections by transmission route.

Table 1. Percentage of Infections by Transmission Route

Route of infection	Percentage of global total
Blood transfusion	3-5
MTCT	5-10
Sexual intercourse	70-80
Injecting drug use	5-10
Health care (needle stick injury, etc.)	<0.01

IMPACTS OF HIV/AIDS

Since the epidemic began, more than 60 million people have been infected with the virus. HIV/AIDS is now by far the leading cause of death in Sub-Saharan Africa, and the fourthbiggest global killer. In 2001, the epidemic claimed about 3 million lives. Some of the manjor impacts of HIV/AIDS are discribed below:

i) *Life expectancy is falling*: In many countries, AIDS is erasing decades of progress made in extending life expectancies. Average life expectancy in Sub-Saharan Africa is now 47 years, when it would have been 62 years without AIDS. Life expectancy at birth in Botswana has dropped to a level not seen in that country since before 1950. In other African countries, life expectancy has dropped less severely, but it is still significantly below what it would have been without AIDS. There is a steep drop in life expectancy in three high prevalence countries, compared to the steady increase in countries with significantly lower HIV prevalence.

   The impact of AIDS on life expectancy, which signifies a major blow to a society's development, has spread beyond Africa. Haiti's life expectancy in 2000–2005 is nearly six years less than it would have been in the absence of AIDS. In Asia, Cambodia has experienced a reduction of four years.

ii) *The death toll rises:* In the 45 most affected countries, it is projected that, between 2000 and 2020, 68 million people will die earlier than they would have in the absence of AIDS. These projections are based on the assumption that prevention, treatment and care programmes will have a modest effect on the growth and impact of the epidemic in most countries over the next two decades. The assumptions do not include a reduction in the annual number of newly infected people, which would result from vaccination with a possible future vaccine or from use of other possible future technological advances. Nor do they include the potential effect of large-scale future access to antiretroviral therapy on the survival of people living with HIV/AIDS.

iii) *The impact on households:* The toll of HIV/AIDS on households can be very severe. In many cases, the presence of AIDS means that the household will dissolve, as parents die and children are sent to relatives for care and upbringing. A study in Zambia revealed that 65 per cent of households in which the mother had died had dissolved. But much happens to a family before this dissolution occurs; HIV/AIDS strips the family of assets and income-earners, further impoverishing those already poor.

iv) *Impact on food security:* HIV/AIDS poses a potentially major threat to food security and nutrition, mainly by diminishing the availability of food (due to falling production, and loss of family labour, land, livestock and other assets) and reducing access to food as households have less money. Researches from Ethiopia has shown that AIDS-affected households were found to spend between 11.6 and 16.4 hours per week performing agricultural work, compared with a mean of 33.6 hours for non-AIDS-affected households.

v) *Impact on the health sector*: In all affected countries, the HIV/AIDS epidemic is bringing additional pressure to bear on the health sector. In countries where per capita health expenditure is low, extending prevention and care for sexually transmitted infections, counselling and testing, prevention of motherto-child transmission services, and HIV treatment and care strains health budgets and systems. As the epidemic matures, the demand for care of those living with HIV/AIDS rises, as does the toll taken among health workers.

vi) *Impact on enterprises and workplaces:* HIV/AIDS dramatically affects labour, setting back economic activity and social progress. The vast majority of people living with HIV/AIDS worldwide are between the ages of 15 and 49— in the prime of their working lives. AIDS weakens economic activity by squeezing productivity, adding costs, diverting productive resources, and depleting skills. In addition, as the impact on households grows more severe, market demand for products and services can shrink. The epidemic hits productivity mainly through increased absenteeism, organisational disruption, and the loss of skills and 'organisational memory'.

vii) *Macroeconomic impact:* Through its impact on the labour force, households and enterprises, HIV/AIDS can act as a significant brake on economic growth and development. Reliable knowledge of the impact of HIV/AIDS on the national economy and its various sectors and participants is valuable for effective national strategic planning and necessary for strong advocacy.

viii) *Security at risk:* AIDS generates more demand for resources and services at all levels of society, while simultaneously weakening the underpinnings of the economy and the State. On the economic and development fronts, several of the worst-affected countries were already struggling with daunting development challenges, excessive debt burdens and declining terms of trade before the epidemic hit. This is most obvious in many sub-Saharan African countries, but is increasingly becoming the case in some countries of the former Soviet Union where socioeconomic setbacks have accompanied economic restructuring. HIV/AIDS is exacerbating these frailties in numerous ways. If effective responses are not introduced and the epidemic is allowed to grow unchecked, its multiple effects could cascade across society, heightening the risk of insecurity, as policymakers are now beginning to discover.

AWARENESS RAISING STRATEGIES

Given the uniquely devastating impact of HIV/AIDS on households, communities and entire societies, national policies and poverty reduction strategies need to be adjusted and expanded accordingly. Unless this happens, AIDS will continue to erode human development achievements, deepen poverty, and further hinder access to education, health and viable livelihoods. However carefully compiled and tallied, data can only hint at the epidemic's human impact, whether at the global, societal, familial or individual level. Mobilising and building the human capacity to cope with, and overcome, the effects of HIV/AIDS is therefore an essential part of an effective response. Often, circumstances have led policymakers and social leaders to enlist community members as leaders of initiatives, rather than positioning them at the receiving end as mere 'beneficiaries' or 'clients'.

Within the education sector, HIV/AIDS has taken its toll on both teachers and pupils.The United Nations (UNICEF, UNESCO, WHO and the World Bank) began the FRESH (Focus Resources on Effective School Health) Partnership, which collaborates with education trade unions affiliated with Education International, ministries of education and teachers' associations, to help strengthen the capacity of teachers to both reduce their own HIV risks and provide HIV/AIDS-related prevention services to their students. Only by directly confronting the issues of teacher shortages and student risks will the two-sided crisis within the education sector be addressed.

The World Health Organisation (WHO) definition of "health" refers to complete physical, mental, spiritual and social well-being, and not merely the absence of disease or infirmity. WHO talks of equity as a prerequisite to achieving the right of good health. Hence, although prevention and treatment are core elements to tackling the disease, it has been argued that greater gains will be made by taking a rights-based approach to tacking HIV/AIDS. This strategy reflects not only the right to good health but also to information and education, freedom of expression and association, liberty and security, privacy and confidentiality, and against inhuman and degrading treatment. This describes a broader more sustainable strategy geared towards improvements in equitable information provision, social reform, infrastructure development and resource mobilisation.

Enhancing Knowledge, Information, Education

Information alone is not enough to change behaviour. It requires effective analysis, communication, participation and accountability to build knowledge and skills. Furthering our understanding of the disease will need to include multidisciplinary assessment of social, economic cultural, behavioural linkages, as well as assessment of policy. Disaggregated data, e.g. by gender, age or income, is crucial to help identify demographic/behavioural trends.

Assessment and collation of examples of good practice is also vital, e.g.,programmes which combine traditional medicinal practice alongside modern medicine, or development of species inventories for traditional medicinal species to help prioritise threatened species and identify the critical habitats which support them. Experimental and clinical evaluation of traditional medicinal plants with anti-rviral, immuno-stimulant and treatment properties is also required, including assessment of their safety and efficacy.

Information resources for education and training programmes should incorporate broad issues such as reproductive and health issues, human rights, abuse, discrimination, biological and cultural aspects. This information needs targeting toward critical groups. For example, young people, of an appropriate age, can be targeted not only at school but more widely, such as in sports and social clubs. The media,e.g., radio, television, theatre, music and the press can also have a powerful impact. Support for parents, carers, policy makers and teachers is vital for community-based outreach to develop awareness amongst peers in schools, families, places of work and recreation.

Enhancing Access to Health Care Services

The right of universal access to "appropriate and affordable" health care services should aim to enhance the ability to choose "safe, effective, affordable and acceptable" methods for family planning, prevention of HIV/AIDS and other STDs, and ensure that services provide a level of care which is affordable, convenient and good quality.

Developing countries clearly need enhanced health care services, including access to voluntary diagnosis and counselling, information and education, referral to alternative services (family planning, confidential diagnosis and treatment), as well as increased research, promotion, supply and distribution of condoms, pharmaceuticals, vaccines and safe blood transfusion. This all requires the mobilisation of considerable resources and skills-sharing within and between countries.

The use of community care plans is increasing, which involves greater support for extended families and community groups,e.g., income and employment generation projects, psychological support and financial assistance, in order to build community capacity to combat the disease. A tiered pricing system for anti-HIV therapies could better reflect the purchasing power parities of different countries to make medicines more affordable. However for the poorest no price is really affordable Mobilisation of external resources are therefore key to help countries obtain and appropriately administer these products.

To enable the rapid adoption and implementation of effective technology, barriers to technology transfer need to be identified. Recently five major drug manufacturers, the WB and UNAIDS met to discuss how to accelerate access and quality of drug provision. Clearly such collaborations should also consider how to accelerating field trials and create incentives for enhancing production and access to medication.

Changing Social Attitudes

If building gender equality and equity is seen as key in the fight against AIDS then changes are necessary in both male and female knowledge, attitudes and behaviour. Women need to develop greater self-esteem and knowledge in order to take more responsibility for their sexual and reproductive health, free from coercion, discrimination, and violence. Men need to take greater responsibility for their own conduct and recognise the importance of women's health and well-being.

To promote gender equality, programmes should highlight the importance of women's health needs and support female involvement in planning, implementation, evaluation and decision making within health provision. Enhancing public acknowledgement and pro-active response to the epidemic will require considerable cultural sensitivity to reflect the diversity of circumstances and needs.

Open discussion, moral and spiritual support for infected and affected people and awareness raising about the disease can help change attitudes and reduce prejudice and discrimination. Publicity campaigns, such as in Brazil, Thailand and Uganda, have shown that a direct link between campaigns, behavioural change and reduced infection. For example an information campaign by the Brazilian Government increased condom use in adults from 5 per cent in 1986 to 50 per cent in 1999. Religious bodies can play a key role in helping to "break the silence" on HIV/AIDS. Many places of worship have initiatives which deal with HIV/AIDS at a local level, e.g., fund raising campaigns, assisting home-based care.

In terms of biological resources, conservation programmes which aim to protect ecosystems are crucial for maintaining known and potential medicinal species. Pharmaceutical companies can incorporate respect for indigenous IPR through royalty and benefit-sharing agreements which may help compensate for use of indigenous knowledge. "Formally" trained practitioners should recognise traditional health practitioners as equals and partnerships encouraged, e.g., through the exchange of information and research which helps to enhance the sustainable conservation, use and management of medicinal plants and their associated ecosystems.

Resource Mobilisation

Improved access, capacity, cost-effectiveness and quality of programmes will require considerable investment. James Wolfensohn, president of the World Bank, recently pledged the maximum available funds to create and implement HIV/ AIDS programmes. One estimate for the global cost of basic health care provision in 2005 was given as $18.5 billion,.7 per cent of which would be for HIV/AIDS related initiatives.

However, more recent UNAIDS figures estimate a total cost between $2-3 billion a year for HIV/AIDS programmes in Africa alone. UNICEF estimates that $2-4 billion will be required to control the epidemic in young people globally (aged 10-15). Increased financial support is needed for research and monitoring, as well as to provide economic support for those infected and affected by HIV/AIDS. Also global and national funds need enhancement to facilitate the transfer and procurement of drugs.

Most funds are expected to come from domestic sources but it is unrealistic to ask many of the developing country governments to meet these costs alone. International initiatives such as the Poverty Reduction Strategy Papers (World Bank) have incorporated facilities targeted to HIV/AIDS programmes in countries such as Nigeria, Mauritania and Burkina Faso. It has also been suggested that domestic resources could be enhanced though debt relief from aid agencies, releasing funds for HIV/AIDS related strategies.

Institutional Roles and Responsibilities

The major roles and responsibilities of various institutions in preventing HIV/AIDS are described below.

Government

a) *Cross departmental response:* enhanced coordination between departments, e.g., labour, defence, education, health, industry, social security. A national AIDS Commission can assist coordination and monitoring of departmental activities.

b) *Promotion of reproductive rights and responsible conduct:* Set up procedures to enable people to report violations of rights and strengthen/enforce laws, e.g., prohibition of child pornography and support gender sensitive strategies that include women at all levels via legislation, policy, projects etc.

c) *Promote community participation:* decentralisation of public health programs, setting up partnerships with focus groups, e.g., local NGOs, women's groups, trade unions, cooperatives, religious groups. Decentralisation requires training and education at more local levels for health care workers, teachers, parents and guardians, and other community representatives.

d) *Resource mobilisation:* Investment in prevention, diagnosis and care is crucial. Rising insurance premiums may not be affordable by employers, thus governments need to encourage policies in the insurance sector which are both affordable and realistic.

e) *Strengthen broad-based health care provision:* Regulate access to health care by establishing standards for diagnosis, drug delivery, patient care and counselling for patients and families. Review international agreementsthat limit access. Create incentives toward better provision, e.g., tax credits to pharmaceutical companies to encourage investment in research where companies are subject to generic competition.

NGOs

a) *Rights based approach:* NGOs, women and community groups, faith communities, etc., can encourage a more equitable approach through greater community interaction e.g. creation of "inter-faith alliances", life-skills training for HIV/AIDS in schools, for organisational members. They can also put pressure on the authorities responsible to provide culturally sensitive and relevant care.

b) *Direct assistance:* NGOs can help implement programmes, through sharing lessons learnt on the ground, assisting exchange of ideas, education and training for community-based prevention and care programs, e.g., through training workshops, conferences, volunteer placements in critical areas.

c) *Protection of Indigenous/traditional knowledge and biological resources:* For example, traditional healers associations can help protect traditional knowledge and conserve biological resources within their native ecosystems, as well as raise community awareness in order to reduce the stigma and risky behaviour associated to infection.

Private sector

a) *Long term business plans*: Work place prevention, care and social investment programs will help save health care costs and enhance labour force productivity, e.g., health education workshops.

b) *Enhancing traditional rights:* Royalty and benefit sharing agreements, partnerships with traditional healers to help protect medicinal species and improve availability and supply of medicinal species through conservation and sustainable harvesting practices.

c) *Safety nets & workers rights:* Pre-employment and on-the job screening can lead to unethical and discriminatory practice, thus the rights of workers need to be incorporated in programmes, e.g., confidential / voluntary testing, equitable insurance and work-related policies.

d) *Business coalitions*: collectively pool resources and response to epidemic, share information on prevention and care, raise awareness in the workplace, e.g., Global Business Council on HIV/AIDS and also national business coalitions in Botswana, Brazil, South Africa and Thailand's have involved trade unions and governments for prompt and effective action against HIV/AIDS.

e) *Awareness raising:* Use of multimedia, e.g., radio, theatre, television, press, music, etc., to reduce stigma, inform people and encourage open debate.

International institutions

a) *Resource mobilisation*: Enhance funding into research for potential species with HIV/AIDS medicinal properties, e.g., Commonwealth Fund for Technical Cooperation.

b) *Advocacy*: Encourage governments, society and other international institutions to set HIV/AIDS as a central development issue and intensify international response, support debt relief and resource mobilisation and expand partnerships, awareness and response.

c) *Access to services and treatment:* Support policies to reduce public sector prices for vaccines and drugs, e.g., UNAIDS "Access to drugs" initiatives in Cote d'Ivoire and Uganda support rational drug selection and use, generic competition and development of national drug management policy. Also International AIDS Vaccine Initiative gives research and technological support for Africa and other developing states. Private sector investment in development of vaccines may be enhanced by procurement of existing vaccines for other diseases, signalling international willingness to pay for AIDS vaccines development. Standardise principles of trade in medicinal plants, e.g., TRAFFIC (Trade Record Analysis of Flora and Fauna in Commerce) guidelines to trade in wildlife (legal and affordable) and clarification of the relevant articles in TRIPS.

d) *Social and cultural rights:* Strengthening of UN goal to eliminate discrimination and violence against women, and provide assistance to victims of any forms of violence in the home, workplace and during armed conflicts. Redefine and monitor IPR to better promote the customary rights of traditional healers, e.g., HARITAF International Working Group on AIDS

e) *Research and information*: Identification of additional needs, e.g. countries in transition. To design, manage and disseminate best practice, technological developments, status reports. Raise the profile of traditional medicine by publishing research findings,

Since UNAIDS was set up, it has made remarkable steps in linking a wide range of actors together, such as setting up the "International Partnership against AIDS in Africa". Largely due to UNAIDS' activities, HIV/AIDS is now on the agenda of many international fora, e.g., the World Education Forum, South Summit, G8 2000 meeting in Japan. At the 13th International AIDS meeting in Durban, the UN Security Council made a resolution recognising HIV/AIDS as an issue of security, linking HIV/AIDS to areas of conflict. Furthermore the UN Economic Commission for Africa decided to focus on AIDS for the African Development Forum in October 2000 and called it *AIDS: the Greatest Leadership Challenge*. These links and on-going discussions need to be maintained and enhanced as what is urgently needed now is action.

UNAIDS advocates localised and national level responses, targeted toward critical groups. Such an approach requires the multi-sectoral involvement of government, pharmaceutical and private sector, academia, women's groups; NGOs, educational institutions, legal and media sectors, as well as those infected with and affected by the disease.

UNAIDS' *Report: on the global HIV/AIDS epidemic* takes the international view a step further by linking the HIV/ AIDS agenda to broader principles of poverty elimination, human rights and sustainable development. Many of the recommendations in UNAIDS' report are focused around International Development Targets agreed upon at various international summits. This includes the specific target of reducing young people's (aged 15-25) vulnerability to HIV/AIDS infection by increasing access to preventative methods (such as condoms, voluntary testing, counselling and follow up) to at least 90 per cent by 2005 and 95 per cent by 2010. In addition the target was set to reduce the rate of HIV infection in young people in "most effected" countries by 25 per cent by 2005 and globally by 2015. It is clear there have been some advancements in meeting these targets. However, strategies need to be continually assessed and reviewed to ensure that they are progressing in the right direction.

HIV/AIDS EDUCATION FOR YOUNG GENERATION

The scale and effects of the HIV/AIDS epidemic were slow to be recognised as a global threat. In response, there have been commendable efforts at international level to capitalise on the potential of formal education as a 'weapon in the fight against HIV'. Both UNICEF and the World Bank emphasise the importance of 'education for all' and increasing general levels of education as a protective measure against HIV. Their stance relies on increasing evidence of a negative correlation between a person's general level of educational attainment and their HIV vulnerability, i.e., the more education a person has, the lower the risk of HIV.

The demographic and health factors such as levels of fertility and life expectancy is linked with education in a number of ways. It is estimated that a one-year increment in mother's education leads to a 7 to 9 per cent decline in under-five mortality. With regards to HIV vulnerability, it is argued that education is correlated with a range of social and cultural factors associated with infection. These include age of sexual debut, age of first marriage, number of children, access to information and culturally specific practices likely to increase vulnerability to HIV, such as wife inheritance and polygamy.

Teaching people how to protect themselves from HIV can lead to a reduction in risk behaviour and hence a reduction in HIV incidence. In response, donors, governments and civil society have rushed into providing HIV/AIDS education as quickly and widely as possible—with school-based HIV/AIDS education being implemented in the vast majority of resource-poor countries. Young people are particularly targeted, because they are seen as a 'window of opportunity' and 'our hope for an AIDS-free generation'. With estimates of 11.8 million young people aged 15 to 24 living with HIV/AIDS it is now vital to understand better how educators are, and should be, responding to the challenges posed by the epidemic.

HIV Education in India and Kenya : Pilot Study of ActionAid

Educational response to the HIV/AIDS epidemic is an important aspect of many social welfare agencies. In this section let us examine the research on HIV education in India and Kenya done by ActionAid, an international NGO.

ActionAid works in partnership with poor communities to fight poverty and its causes. ActionAid's recognition, 15 years ago, that HIV/AIDS was a significant threat to the development of poor countries, has led to pioneering work in prevention, community-based care and advocacy, including developing the Stepping Stones methodology and supporting community-based organisations, such as TASO in Uganda. Its work concentrates on encouraging and supporting local innovation and action and trying to change the global political and social structures that make poor communities vulnerable. ActionAid works with local partners in 15 African and four Asian countries to ensure that people and communities affected by HIV/AIDS are at the centre of developing effective responses to the epidemic.

In the first few months of 2002 ActionAid offices in Tanzania, Malawi and Kenya each carried out small-scale pieces of research into how education is affected by HIV/AIDS.

Although the methodology varied between the countries, each research team attempted to assess the opinions of local communities on two distinct but interrelated topics: (i) how HIV/AIDS education is being communicated, and (ii) how schooling has changed as a consequence of increasing prevalence rates of HIV.

The main research took place in India and Kenya during the summer of 2002. ActionAid offices in these countries had already identified HIV/AIDS education as an issue of concern. It was decided to undertake a situational analysis and to identify key policy and programme positions – to inform work in the individual countries and to contribute to wider learning across ActionAid as a whole. As the epidemic is at different stages of advance in the two countries, the study also offered the opportunity to meet one of ActionAid's priorities, that poor communities should learn from each other and, in particular, that Asia should learn from African experiences of HIV/AIDS.

The research is aimed to answer the following questions:

i) What is the expressed demand for HIV/AIDS education by young people, parents and their communities?
ii) What is thought to be the role of the school in meeting the above demand?
iii) How do students and parents perceive the way that HIV/AIDS is taught in school?
iv) What are the difficulties identified by teachers and students, and how might they be overcome?

Fieldwork was conducted during June 2002 in Kenya and July/August 2002 in India. Learning from the Kenya research was used to fine-tune the research tools and methodology used in India.

The research was conducted in Nyanza province, Kenya, and Tamil Nadu state, India. In both countries the selected areas have higher than average national HIV/AIDS prevalence rates. Also of importance for the research, each region has implemented a programme of HIV education in state schools.

In Nyanza province, research took place in one rural setting (Homa Bay) and one urban setting (Kisumu). The main industries are fishing and agriculture; the main ethnic group is the Luo, the third largest ethnic group in Kenya. About 90 per cent of the population is Christian, although traditional beliefs are still common.

Nyanza province is one of the poorest provinces in Kenya. According to the Demographic and Health Survey, (DHS) 1998, a substantial proportion of the population in Nyanza has no access to mass media, particularly women. The median age of marriage in the province is 17.5 years for women with sexual debut averaging at 15.6 years. HIV prevalence rates are amongst the highest in Kenya with about one in three pregnant women testing positive at antenatal clinics in the region – this is over double the national prevalence of 15 per cent and the area is probably one of the highest sero-prevalence regions in the world. The main mode of HIV transmission is identified as being through heterosexual intercourse. A recent UNAIDS study which included Kisumu suggested that a number of factors increased vulnerability to HIV: reported behavioural factors included young age at first marriage for women, and a considerable age difference between spouses.

According DHS, 1998, at 73.5 per cent, literacy is relatively high in the state though, as in other parts of India, female literacy is substantially lower than male. Women in the state marry much younger than men, the median ages being 20.9 and 26.6 respectively; 24 per cent of young women aged 15 to 19 years are married, with the number rising significantly in rural areas. Urban areas have more access to communications –only 9 per cent of people in urban areas have no access to mass media, compared to over 25 per cent of those living in rural areas.

According to the National AIDS Control Organisation's report, 2002, HIV prevalence among women visiting antenatal clinics in Tamil Nadu is around 1.1 per cent, one of the highest in the country.

A combination of quantitative and qualitative approaches was employed for the research. The main research tools were:

i) self-completion, structured questionnaires for parents and students
ii) interviewer-administered questionnaires amongst parents
iii) individual semi-structured interviews with head-teachers and other key informants
iv) focus group discussions with students (India and Kenya) and teachers (India only).

Each of the interviews explored aspects of the HIV syllabus and asked respondents what they thought about HIV/AIDS education. Questions covered four main areas:

i) demand for HIV/AIDS education
ii) the role of schools in meeting that demand
iii) policy and practice of HIV/AIDS education
iv) overcoming difficulties in teaching HIV/AIDS education.

Individual interviews and focus group discussions were designed to probe on specific issues emerging from the quantitative stage and to achieve deeper understanding of respondents' answers. Interviewing was conducted by teams of researchers and supervisors in each country under the guidance of Amina Ibrahim in Kenya and Ranjin Adoss in India. Table 1 summarises the composition of the survey sample. It was not intended that these findings would be representative of the total populations of the countries in question, more that they would be indicative of the views of communities experiencing relatively high levels of HIV and which have been exposed to some form of school-based education on the topic.

It was the purpose of the research to include sufficient interviews to produce significant results for key segments – that is, gender, school stage and geographic location and to allow for comparisons between the groups of greatest interest in each

Table 2. Summary of interviews achieved

Area	Schools	Student questionnaire (self–completion)	Teacher questionnaire (self–completion)	Parent questionnaire (interviewer administered)	Qualitative phase	Key informant interviews
Kenya						
(Nyanza province)		1,198	291	291	30 student focus group discussions	Curriculum design
Kisumu district (urban)	20 primary					AIDS control organisations
Homa Bay district (rural)	10 primary				30 headteacher interviews	Teacher training
						Education officers
India						Community leaders
(Tamil Nadu)						Religious leaders
Chenna (urban)	30 schools all secondary	1,201	299	299	42 student focus group discussions	NGOs
	10 High Schools (X)					
Tuticorin (rural)	10 Higher Secondary (XI)					34 interviews in total
	10 Higher Secondary (XII)				30 headteacher interviews	
					20 teacher focus group discussions	

country. One urban and one rural area were chosen in each state and interviews were evenly split between these. In Nyanza these included primary and secondary schools (as HIV/AIDS education is taught from Standard 1 of primary school). In Tamil Nadu, only high school and higher secondary schools were sampled because HIV/AIDS education is not introduced into the syllabus until Standard 8 of secondary school.

More purposive sampling was used in India, which included a mixture of state and private, Hindu, Christian and Muslim schools, to allow some comparison across schools. In Kenya, all were government schools. In India, students were evenly split between those studying science subjects and those studying arts subjects.

For each school:

— An interview was conducted with the school principal/headteacher.

— The teacher questionnaire was administered to a maximum of ten teachers in each school, including all those involved in HIV/AIDS education plus a selection teaching other subjects. A range of age and gender was included. In India, all of the teachers directly involved in teaching about HIV & AIDS were also asked to participate in a focus group discussion. Alternatively, individual or paired depth interviews took place depending on individual school circumstances.

— Students from each year group were randomly chosen (gender–balanced) and asked to complete questionnaires.

— After completing the questionnaire, a group of five to eight students (of the same sex) from one of the age groups was randomly chosen (but balanced across the total sample) and asked to stay behind for a focus group discussion. Each group lasted for around one hour.

— Additionally, parents with children in the year groups being researched (though not necessarily parents of the actual student respondents) were invited to take part in an interviewer-administered questionnaire. A target was set of 12 parent interviews per school. Across the whole sample an even gender and student year group split was achieved.

— Key stakeholder interviews were conducted in the locale or in regional/national offices where appropriate.

Bilingual interviewers and moderators were used in both countries, though the Kenyan research team preferred to use materials in English whilst the Indian team opted for Tamil versions. All questionnaires and interview notes were transcribed into English in country, but were processed and analysed in the UK.

Permission was obtained from education authorities to interview in the selected schools. Additional permission was sought from parents to speak with children. High levels of privacy were maintained whilst respondents were participating in the research and guarantees of anonymity were given.

Individual interviews and focus group discussions were tape recorded and transcribed where permission was given. Otherwise notes were taken. Where possible moderators were the same sex as participants. Small incentives were provided to all survey respondents. Data analysis was carried out in the UK by Vital Statistics, a specialist data processing agency.

Demand for HIV/AIDS education

One of the key aims of the research was to find out what level of support HIV/AIDS education has at the community level—this ties in strongly with ActionAid's approach of working in partnership with communities. Research suggests that community resistance to young people being taught about HIV does exist—and can lead to teacher anxiety of potential criticism from parents.

It seems clear from both the quantitative and qualitative research that most parents, students and teachers view HIV/AIDS education as important and necessary: 69 per cent of

Indian teachers and 80 per cent of Kenyan teachers said that it was very important to have HIV/AIDS education in schools. Attitudes vary according to the perceived extent of the problem and what should and should not be taught.

Parental knowledge of HIV/AIDS curriculum: Parents were asked if they were aware that their children were being taught about HIV/AIDS in school: 68 per cent of Kenyan parents said they were, compared to only 12 per cent of Indian parents. There were striking urban and rural differences in each country. Parents in rural areas reported having significantly less knowledge of HIV/AIDS education than their urban counterparts—82 per cent of Indian respondents in rural areas reported knowing 'not much' about HIV/AIDS education in schools, compared to 27 per cent in urban areas. In Kenya, the comparative figures were 40 per cent in rural areas and 21 per cent in urban areas.

Parental attitudes towards HIV/AIDS education : In order to gauge what attitudes parents had towards their children learning about HIV/AIDS in school, parents and teachers were asked to state their level of agreement that: 'on the whole, parents in this school want their children to be taught about HIV/AIDS.' Overall, the vast majority of parents said that they did want their children to learn about HIV/AIDS. The interesting dynamic is that most teachers perceive parental support to be lower than it is. Additional interviews with parents and teachers seem to support this finding. While teachers often feared a backlash from angry parents, the majority of parents in both countries said they were supportive of HIV/AIDS education.

The discordance between teacher and parent perceptions is larger in India than Kenya: teachers in India seem to be less confident of parental support than their Kenyan counterparts. In India, interviews supported the idea that teachers' fear of criticism was the result of parents directly making complaints to the school. It is important, however, to keep in mind that the majority of teachers in both countries (55 per cent in India;

63 per cent in Kenya) thought that there was parental support for HIV/AIDS education. Many students also claimed that their parents wanted them to learn about HIV.

Teachers can rely on the support of the parents and communities in teaching HIV/AIDS. Although this support does exist, it seems that a minority of parents with strong opposition to HIV/AIDS education have overly influenced teachers' judgement. Strengthening links between the school and the community is one way of increasing parental support of HIV/AIDS education. No school exists in a vacuum and, especially in the case of HIV/AIDS, education has the potential to extend out into the community and make a difference. These links could be created through parent-teacher associations, school-home liaison or through community-based organisations.

Perceived risk to HIV/AIDS

In trying to understand parental attitudes towards HIV/AIDS education, it is important to also understand general attitudes towards the size of the problem and the extent to which parents think their children are at risk. Respondents were asked if they viewed HIV/AIDS as a problem that touches upon their personal lives, and what they perceived the level of risk behaviour to be in their school.

Respondents were asked how serious a problem they viewed HIV/AIDS to be at different levels: in the world, their country, their local area and their school. There were strong levels of agreement between parents, teachers and students in both countries.

The epidemic in India is usually identified as being at an early stage, and compared to many Sub-Saharan countries, prevalence rates are relatively low. However, the majority of students, parents and teachers in both countries viewed HIV/AIDS to be a very big problem in their own country. In India, respondents reported that HIV/AIDS was not such a big problem in their local area – an interesting finding as prevalence rates in Tamil Nadu are among the highest in the country.

In general people do not personalise HIV/AIDS as a problem but see it as something that only happens to other people in other places. They do not therefore see themselves as personally at risk. Knowledge and awareness are not enough to reduce risk behaviour and that perceptions of personally being susceptible must also exist. Perceived threat involves two components: perceived risk and perceived severity. This idea is supported by some of the interviews in both countries, which show that having actual personal experience of HIV/AIDS is important in order to perceive risk. Many interviews show underlying assumptions of 'us' and 'them', with the blame for some 'morally deplorable behaviour' being firmly placed on 'them'.

The vast majority of respondents in Nyanza claimed HIV/AIDS to be a very big problem in their local area. This makes sense: adult prevalence is estimated to be over 30 per cent. HIV in Nyanza is much more personal, and approximately three out of ten students reported the death of their fathers, compared to only 10 per cent of Indian students. As most of Kenyan parents in the sample were aged below 44 (61 per cent), it can be assumed that this degree of adult mortality within these age ranges is caused by HIV/AIDS. Clearly, HIV/AIDS has directly affected the lives of many of the Kenyan students who responded to the survey.

In Kenya, perceptions of the size of the problem in schools differ between respondents; 67 per cent of teachers and 73 per cent of parents view HIV/AIDS to be a very big problem in their school, while less than half of the students (42 per cent) agree. This may explain a common theme in the interviews with teachers, who often complained that students viewed HIV as something that would not personally affect them, only 'others'.

An overly scientific approach to HIV/AIDS education risks being divorced from any reality which young people can relate to. Having some form of human connection is helpful in understanding HIV and personal risk.

To communicate effectively with young people on a sensitive issue like HIV may require a different pedagogy to that associated with traditional learning in the classroom. Although teachers should be encouraged to broaden their own pedagogic base, there is also great potential in involving or developing external resource groups. Governments could encourage the formation or strengthening of mobile groups, such as those that use theatre, song, dance or storytelling, which can be supported to tour around schools in each district. Specific incentives may be offered to such groups whether at national or district level for them to develop work on HIV/AIDS and make links with schools.

The use of different forms of creative communication can humanise HIV/AIDS, bringing home key messages more powerfully than merely reading from textbooks. Positive speakers may be invited to schools to talk about living positively with HIV. Not only will these speakers help to add that crucial human element, they will also help break down stigma and discrimination, as young people see that it is possible to live positively with HIV. It is also important for young people to see that people with HIV often look healthy as it is a common misconception that you can tell by looking at someone if they have HIV or not.

Perceived risk behaviour in school

The questionnaire asked about the frequency of a small number of possible risk behaviours; casual sexual relationships; pregnancies (as proxy for unprotected sexual intercourse); and use of alcohol and drugs. Respondents in both countries were asked how frequently occurring they perceived each of these to be. In Kenya there is an acceptance that these relationships are taking place—quite opposite to the view from India.

Similar trends were found when respondents were asked about pregnancy, alcohol and drugs. Indian and Kenyan respondents showed opposite patterns of response, but there was generally strong agreement between students, parents and teachers within each country. For example, on the issue of pregnancy, 78 per cent of Kenyan teachers and 70 per cent of parents said it happens sometimes or a lot whilst in India, 80 per cent of Indian students and parents and 77 per cent of teachers said that it never happens.

In Nyanza, risk behaviours within the school—such as casual and unprotected sex—were reported by the majority of students, with only a minority reporting that these behaviours never happen.

In Tamil Nadu the opposite appears to be true, with the majority of all respondents saying these risk behaviours never happen. In interviews many of the teachers explained that there was a high level of control exerted over young people, both by the school and their parents.

Many of the other interviews also suggested that male and female students in Tamil Nadu's mixed-gender schools are segregated to the extent that they not only sit in separate parts of the classroom, but are forbidden to talk to each other.

For perceived levels of risk behaviour to affect the demand for HIV/AIDS education, parents and teachers would need to view these behaviours as (i) a problem (ii) being related to HIV (iii) influenced by education.

i) *Kenyan teachers' perceptions of student behaviour:* Many teachers in Kenya clearly thought that student behaviour was a problem.
ii) *Behaviour related to HIV vulnerability:* Pregnancy is one of the clearest indications of unprotected sex. Not only are student pregnancies linked to HIV but that they are also linked to low levels of HIV/AIDS education. If the students had more HIV/AIDS education there would be less unprotected sex and that education can and will lead to behaviour change.
iii) *Education for behaviour change:* Most health education theories are founded on the belief that education is a necessary component to realising behaviour change. As

mentioned earlier, the Health Belief model suggests that some element of knowledge and awareness is needed.

The empirical data, in particular the more behaviouralist interpretations of behaviour change, indicate that education is necessary but not sufficient to reduce risk behaviour. In India, in the context of a more recently acknowledged epidemic, the findings from the interviews suggest there is a strong belief that educating students about the dangers of HIV will protect them in the future. In contrast, Kenyan respondents were more sceptical—perhaps after having experienced a more severe epidemic, more HIV/AIDS education, and less observed behaviour change.

Young people need more than knowledge – they also need the skills to apply that knowledge to everyday situations which are far removed from the classroom. In addition to skills, people need the power to leverage their sexual health rights. One critical element of ActionAid's work in both the fields of education and HIV has been to challenge ingrained gender and power relations which contribute to the rapid spreading of the HIV/AIDS epidemic. Examining gender inequality and its effect on communication in sexual relationships needs to be cardinal to any education approach which truly aims to change sexual behaviour. The challenge is to find constructive ways to work with men as well as women, and boys as well as girls, to address the wider gender and power issues that affect communication within sexual relationships.

Perceived responsibility of HIV/AIDS education

The research suggests that there is a demand for HIV/AIDS education in both Tamil Nadu and Nyanza. To consider the question of responsibility, teachers were asked who should teach children about HIV. They were asked to tick as many categories as appropriate. There are striking differences between responses in Kenya and India. Although the most common answer for both countries was teachers, in Kenya, responsibility is perceived to be much more spread out, and incorporates the whole spectrum from parents to religious leaders to government— perhaps out of recognition of the need for a multi-sectoral response. In India, most of the perceived responsibility lies with the teacher.

Parents, teachers and students were asked where they thought young people learnt about HIV/AIDS. The questionnaire included 20 possible categories, and respondents were asked to tick as many as appropriate and then list the three sources they considered to be most important. There was a high level of consistency between respondents' answers in each country. Similar to other research, the findings suggest that there are a number of social influences on young people.

Role of mass media: In both Kenya and India, television was rated as one of the top three sources of information by all respondents. However, although mass media is clearly an important source of information for young people, it may be less so for young women than it is for men.

In India television is often viewed as a negative influence. Some respondents expressed concern that the information is unsuitable and could lead to sexual experimentation. The role of the school is therefore prioritised because of its potential to counterbalance 'misinformation' from television. The majority of Indian respondents did not cite any family member as a source of information.

In contrast, the majority of Kenyan respondents listed all family members, especially the mother. Female students in both countries were more likely than their male counterparts to report learning about HIV/AIDS from their mothers: 17 per cent of female Indian students as opposed to 6 per cent of males; 78 per cent of Kenyan females compared to 69 per cent of males.

Kenyan parents appear to talk to their children about sex and HIV/AIDS far more than Indian parents. When asked why they did not talk to their children about such issues, 31 per cent of Indian parents said because they did not like to talk about sex.

Role of the family: The role of the family in HIV/AIDS education seems to differ greatly between India and Kenya. The data indicates clearly that the family, particularly the mother, is more open in talking about HIV/AIDS and sex to their children in Nyanza compared to Tamil Nadu. Female students are also more likely to learn about HIV/AIDS from their mothers than male students.

In Tamil Nadu there were strong differences between urban and rural areas, with parents in rural areas much less likely to discuss sex or HIV/AIDS with their children: 82 per cent of parents in Tuticorin claimed never to have talked to their child about sex or HIV/AIDS compared to 44 per cent of respondents in Chennai.

In both countries, perceived difficulties for parents to talk to their children about HIV/AIDS was implicitly given as a rationale for the school to teach HIV/AIDS. In Kenya the extended family newtork also appears to play an important role in teaching young people about sensitive issues such as HIV.

Role of religious leaders: Kenyan respondents were far more likely than Indian respondents to list religious leaders as a source of HIV/AIDS information. In addition, a significant percentage of Kenyan respondents listed religious leaders as one of the top three sources of information (14 per cent of students, 17 per cent of teachers and 11 per cent of parents).

Peer influence: A high percentage of respondents in both Kenya (70 per cent) and India (43 per cent) reported learning about HIV/AIDS from friends. Interestingly, there was also a strong gender dynamic in India, where 52 per cent of male Indian students cited their friends as somewhere they get information on HIV, compared to 33 per cent of female students. In addition, 20 per cent of male students listed friends as one of their top three sources of information, compared to 8 per cent of female students. It is not clear from the research whether peer influence is either negative or positive. The interviews showed rather mixed responses on this issue. In Kenya there was significant reporting of negative peer influence which was not so apparent in India.

The large number of potential sources of information on HIV is problematic in that it increases the probability of young people receiving conflicting messages. Although teachers in Nyanza did not discuss any negative impact of mass media, 50 per cent viewed contradictory information as a barrier to delivering HIV/AIDS education, compared to only 18 per cent of Indian teachers. However, conflicting information does not only come from the media. In Kenya, it is likely that contradictory messages also come from traditional healers or religious leaders: 29 per cent of Kenyan teachers viewed religious teachings as barriers to HIV/AIDS education, compared to 7 per cent of Indian teachers.

Policy Framework for HIV/AIDS Education

Sexual and reproductive health education has been a contentious issue for some time, even before HIV and AIDS were discovered. Key issues concern whether or not teaching young people (who are not yet sexually active) about sex will lead to increased sexual experimentation, and how the subject should be taught: either 'fact based' (the scientific approach) and/or 'skill based' (the life skills approach).

When HIV and AIDS first became part of school curricula, emphasis was placed on topics such as the structure of the virus or what happens to the body after infection. Early approaches tried to instil as much scientific fact about HIV/AIDS as possible. This approach was based on the assumption that increasing levels of knowledge and awareness would lead to the desired behaviour change.

Having accurate information about how the virus is passed is undoubtedly a necessary part of protecting oneself against the virus, however, it is not sufficient. Young people must also have the necessary skills to apply their knowledge. This realisation has led to a move to a more life skills approach, teaching a wide range of skills which go beyond HIV. The rather broad definition by World Health Organisation is as follows:

> Life skills are abilities for adaptive and positive behaviour that enable individuals to deal effectively with the demands and challenges of everyday life.

Three equally broad categories of skills that would apply to the life skills approach include:

i) communication and interpersonal skills
ii) decision-making and critical thinking skills
iii) coping and self-management skills

School curricula on HIV will differ according to the extent to which they tackle the issues from a scientific approach, or a life skills approach. A combination of both approaches would reduce the limitations that arise in using one approach exclusively. The shift to a life skills approach goes some way to meeting some of the criticisms that simply increasing awareness will not lead to behaviour change.

HIV/AIDS curricula: The HIV/AIDS curricula in Kenya and India differ greatly. The curriculum was introduced in Kenya in 2000—one year after HIV/AIDS was officially declared a national disaster. HIV/AIDS education was added to the curriculum as a separate subject which took the place of a physical education (PE) class, and is typically taught by PE teachers for half an hour a week. The syllabus starts from Standard 1 of primary school. The curriculum is broad and deals with both scientific aspects of the disease and the more social and cultural factors.

The government provides facilitators' handbooks for teachers. As of yet, there is no official training on how to implement the curriculum, although Nyanza has participated in a pilot training study run jointly by DFID and the Kenyan Government. In addition to this separate subject, HIV/AIDS is integrated and infused across the curriculum.

In Tamil Nadu, lessons on HIV/AIDS have been included in the syllabus for Tamil, English, botany, zoology and science.

The lessons are more scientific than in Kenya, covering issues such as the structure of the HIV virus or disease progression. In addition, these lessons are only available to science students after Standard 10.

School-based HIV/AIDS education is limited in scope because of its failure to reach the millions of children who are not currently in the formal education system. There are estimated to be more than 115 million children out of school worldwide. These children are likely to come from more vulnerable sectors of society and are potentially more at risk of HIV infection than young people who are in the formal education system.

Moreover, if school-based HIV/AIDS education does not start until secondary school, then even more children will be excluded. This is the case in India, where more than half of young people never even enrol in secondary school and therefore have limited access to HIV/AIDS information compared to their counterparts who are in school.

In Kenya, over 70 per cent of children never reach secondary school. To ensure that all young people are reached by HIV/AIDS education, there must be either a massive increase in the percentage of youth participating in the formal education system or else, schools should seriously consider how HIV/AIDS learning in the classroom could extend back into the community. More recently there has been the introduction of the Total Health Programme, funded by UNICEF, which has a much wider scope, but does include HIV.

Very limited research has been devoted to the implementation of HIV/AIDS education in the classroom. A qualitative study in Uganda suggested that teachers were reluctant to teach about condoms and also avoided the more 'participatory' elements of the curriculum. Similarly, some anecdotal evidence suggests that teachers actively shy away from teaching HIV/AIDS.

It is important to know how HIV/AIDS is being taught in the classroom and what messages are being given out to young people. In order to gain some rough indication of how HIV/AIDS was being taught in the classroom, the questionnaires asked students to list topics on the curriculum that had been taught. One of the limitations of the research was that it was carried out in the middle of the school year, therefore, for some either the curriculum hadn't been covered yet or else students had forgotten because it was covered some time ago.

Selective teaching: Some students claimed that the lessons as laid out in the syllabus were simply not being taught at all. In Tamil Nadu, 95 per cent of teachers claimed the Total Health Programme was being taught, but only 53 per cent of students agreed: If the Total Health Programme is not being taught in Tamil Nadu, this is not a case of omitting certain topics, but an entire curricular subject.

In Nyanza, all schools are supposed to have started HIV/AIDS education. However, 8 per cent of the Kenyan students said that they had never been taught about HIV in school. In both Kenya and India, reports of selective teaching was higher in rural than urban areas. For instance, in India, only 46 per cent of students in rural areas reported having been taught the Total Health Programme compared to 60 per cent in urban areas.

The quantitative analysis shows some level of selective teaching: there are several strong links between what teachers consider to be important to teach and how much students say they have been taught. For example, in Kenya, 'beliefs and practices which affect the spread of HIV/AIDS' was rated as the least important topic to teach by teachers. Students claimed that this was the least taught topic on the syllabus: 59 per cent of students claimed it was being taught, compared to 91 per cent for responsible behaviour and 93 per cent for transmission of HIV. These findings suggest that the syllabus is being taught selectively, a conclusion that was reinforced in some of the focus group discussions with students. Some teachers seem to avoid teaching lessons which are sensitive and, perhaps, embarrassing. This would also explain why the topic on cultural practices and beliefs is being missed out, as it is less straightforward and more sensitive than other more scientific topics.

Teachers appear to be teaching some lessons on HIV, but exercising their own judgement in which messages should be taught and which not. There are likely to be two reasons for this:

i) difficulties in discussing sex, leading to discussions of HIV without talking about sex
ii) societal and religious pressures that forbid the discussion of safer sex, leading to HIV/AIDS lessons which emphasise abstinence without raising issues on safe sex.

In the context of AIDS epidemics which are being spread mostly through heterosexual intercourse in both Tamil Nadu and Nyanza, a discussion on HIV/AIDS without talking about sex will be inherently limited. Most models which relate education to behaviour change rely on some premise of awareness of risk. It is impossible to have a clear idea of personal levels of risk to the virus without knowledge of how HIV is, and is not, transmitted. Despite this, sex is such a taboo subject in many countries that there is high resistance to opening such a discussion. In both countries a significant percentage of students had had HIV/AIDS education without ever having had any lessons on sex.

HIV/AIDS education without direct reference to sex appears to be much more common in Tamil Nadu than Nyanza: approximately one-third of the Indian students reported having had lessons on HIV/AIDS but not sex, compared to only 7 per cent of the Kenyan students. The reason for this is probably the emphasis in Tamil Nadu on teaching HIV/AIDS as a scientific subject, extracting sex and human relations from the equation. A common thread running through the Indian interviews was the underlying belief that HIV/AIDS consisted of scientific fact and should be taught accordingly, and any other way of teaching could lead to sexual experimentation and raise passions.

More female students reported having had lessons on HIV/AIDS and sex in rural and urban areas of both countries. For instance, 60 per cent of female Indian students claimed to have had lessons on sex, compared to 54 per cent of their male counterparts. The reason for this trend is not clear. It is possible that, for gender-specific reasons, female students are actually receiving more sex education. Alternatively, there may be a gender bias in the reporting, with female respondents perhaps being more open about having received sex education. Teachers also expressed concern that parents would disapprove if they knew that the students were being taught about sex.

In Kenya, something different appears to be happening. HIV/AIDS education involves more lessons which include sex education than India, but the messages on sex are highly selective. HIV/AIDS education gives people strong messages on appropriate and safe sexual behaviour. The three key messages used around the world are: (a) abstain (b) be faithful and (c) use condoms. However, there is controversy over whether or not the 'C' component should be taught at all. Roth examined condom use in India and concluded that the cultural and social climate renders "the existing educational and disease prevention strategies inappropriate and ineffective". In this quote he is referring specifically to the promotion of condoms and safe sex. Certain religious institutions are also against the teaching of the 'C' component with the Vatican probably being the most vocal in its stance against condoms. Although it has not been shown empirically, it has been suggested that religious barriers that oppose the promotion of condoms lead to ineffective prevention strategies. In his study in the Masaka district of Uganda, Kinsman suggested that there were four interrelated factors which deterred teachers from discussing condoms in the classroom:

i) the belief that condoms will encourage promiscuity,
ii) the influence of the Roman Catholic church,

iii) fear that the headteacher will fire the teacher, and

iv) personal beliefs of teachers.

The research aimed to examine how teachers in the two countries view condoms and what messages about sex are being given out in school-based HIV/AIDS education. In both countries, there was a strong belief that refraining from any sexual relationship is the best, and the only way to stop the further spread of HIV. There was also the belief that educating young people about methods of safer sex will lead to sexual experimentation. In the questionnaire respondents were asked whether or not they thought students should have access to condoms, as a way to gauge their opinions towards safer sex and condoms. There was strong resistance towards condoms in both countries and amongst all categories of respondents. Students in both countries were more likely to agree to access to condoms than their parents and teachers. The findings also show that there was less disagreement towards access in Tamil Nadu than Nyanza. In Kenya, respondents were more certain of their negative stance towards condoms: 57 per cent of Kenyan respondents disagreed strongly, compared to 28 per cent in India. One likely reason is the strong influence of the Roman Catholic church in Nyanza and its stance against condoms.

The Catholic Church appears to exert a strong influence on HIV/AIDS education in Nyanza. Religious influence in Tamil Nadu doesn't appear to be as strong, certainly in the state sector. 22 per cent of students in Nyanza reported having learnt about HIV during religious teachings. Also, more Kenyan students, teachers and parents said that religious leaders supported HIV/AIDS education in school than their Indian counterparts.

Although the results suggest stronger religious support of in HIV/AIDS education in Kenya than India, a significant proportion of teachers in both countries viewed religious leaders not to be supportive: a significant proportion of teachers in both countries viewed religious teachings to act as a barrier to HIV/AIDS education, particularly in Kenya.

HIV/AIDS education should acknowledge the influence of the religious institutions and look at how to involve and include local spiritual leaders. It is important that there is consistency in the messages given on HIV/AIDS between schools and church. Religious leaders need to be brought together and asked how they will respond to the human crisis which has arisen because of HIV. Their role in educating young people about HIV and condoms must be used positively. However, religious leaders cannot be expected to have the knowledge and skills needed to discuss HIV openly, accurately and positively. If not, there will be contradictions between the messages received by young people at school and in church. Contradictions lead to confusion and can propagate potentially negative myths. Myths and misconceptions about condoms, such as the one above, are potentially very damaging. It is important to know what myths are being circulated among young people and then to challenge them.

Paradox of safer sex education: It is worrying that safer sex is not being taught to students, precisely because the findings show that risky sexual behaviour is perceived to be fairly common in Kenyan schools. Evidence from a recent study in Kisumu showed that reported condom use was highest amongst those with the most knowledge of HIV. HIV/AIDS education which addresses the issue of condoms can lead to safer sexual practices.

The paradox of safer sex arises from a tension between two assumptions that fit ill with one another. One is an assumption that students might be having sex, and therefore HIV is a genuine risk; the necessary assumption to discuss condoms. The other is what might be call as a 'societal assumption', which results from deep-seated social pressures. In this case the societal assumption is 'we do not and will not have pre-marital sex'. Clearly they are contradictory, and the paradox of safer sex arises precisely because both find themselves thrust upon the educational agenda, the first by the HIV/AIDS curriculum and the second by deeply entrenched societal pressures.

Accepting condoms as a method of reducing the risk of HIV must assume that young people are having, or might have, pre-marital sex. However, this can contradict deeply ingrained societal assumptions that pre-marital sex doesn't happen. It therefore becomes rationally impossible to discuss safer sex. Resolving the tension in this paradox means dropping one of the above assumptions. Assuming that students will not have pre-marital sex is a familiar response: 'HIV isn't our problem—it happens to others, to immoral sorts'. This assumption leads to stigma and discrimination, and in refusing to acknowledge the problem, there is little hope of solving it. Only an effort to challenge the 'societal assumption', in this case that sex before marriage does not happen, is likely to bring about any real change. This means challenging the cultural assumptions of the societies in which HIV is prevalent. It is hard, but not impossible. However, challenging a country's social norms carries the threat of cultural imperialism—especially if outsiders are perceived to be challenging or, more often than not, criticising. Moreover, it is paramount that positive social norms are not undermined.

Obstacles to teaching HIV/AIDS

Teachers are hampered in their efforts to teach HIV/AIDS in the classroom for a number of reasons, including low prioritisation of HIV/AIDS education, and material factors such as insufficient learning materials. Qualitative research using focus group discussions suggested that teachers found it difficult to teach about HIV in Zambia, because of a lack of training and insufficient learning materials.

Despite huge international mobilisation to provide universal primary education, in many countries formal education systems are under duress. Although there have been commendable increases in enrolment in many countries, these increases have unfortunately been accompanied by decreases in quality.

The quality of formal education systems in resource-poor settings has been eroded over the years through chronic under-financing. The resource gap for providing universal primary education currently stands at $5.6 billion per year. Moreover, The large number of out-of-school children, which is symptomatic of the wider crisis in education, also has huge implications for school-based HIV/AIDS education by significantly limiting its scope.

Systematic progress towards quality education for all is generally measured using two proxies: (i) educational expenditures and (ii) pupil-teacher ratios.

i) *Educational expenditure*: The EFA monitoring report estimates India to have resource gaps of between 1 and 4 billion dollars per year – this is the level of additional investment needed to reach international targets of universal primary education by 2015. In Kenya, estimates are between 70 and 172 million dollars per year.
ii) *Pupil–teacher ratios:* As a general indicator of the underlying quality of education in Tamil Nadu and Nyanza, teachers were asked to indicate average class sizes.

Over 40 per cent of classes in the Indian sample averaged at over 50 students. With classes this large, it is questionable how much learning can take place, and the quality of education each student receives is seriously undermined. In Kenya, teacher shortages are being compounded by the HIV/AIDS epidemic.

Teachers were asked what difficulties they faced in teaching HIV/AIDS. On the whole, Kenyan teachers cited a much larger number of obstacles than their Indian counterparts. However, the three obstacles most commonly cited in both countries were the same.

Table 3

Most commonly cited obstacles in teaching HIV/AIDS

Most commonly cited obstacles	*India*	*Kenya*
1.	Lack of resources	Lack of resources
2.	Cultural barriers	Lack of training
3.	Lack of training	Cultural barriers
4.	Parental resistance	Contradictory information

Learning resources: Lack of learning materials was one of the most commonly cited barriers to HIV/AIDS education by teachers in both countries; 62 per cent of students in Kenya said their schools did not have enough teaching materials to teach about HIV/AIDS, compared to 67 per cent of Indian students. A massive injection of resources is needed in order to support teachers – not just for teaching about HIV/AIDS, but to ensure some modicum of quality education for all.

Teachers' levels of knowledge: All respondents were asked if they thought teachers had enough knowledge to teach HIV/AIDS. Although the majority of respondents in both countries perceived teachers to have enough knowledge to teach HIV/AIDS, overall confidence in teachers' competence appears lower in Kenya than India. The pattern of differences between respondents was similar for the two countries – both parents and students reported having more confidence in teachers' levels of knowledge than the teachers themselves. This interpretation is consistent with the idea that both students and parents were shifting responsibility for HIV/AIDS education onto the teachers and that this might be a leap of faith, as the teachers themselves are not as confident about their abilities.

One way of increasing levels of knowledge is to provide distance-learning materials for teachers. These could include training manuals, videos or interactive learning modules. However, as discussed above, learning materials are already in short supply. Many schools would not have the facilities to use electronic materials, even if they were easily available. Moreover, learning materials alone will not equip teachers with the skills to teach confidently about HIV/AIDS and sex—they also need practical training.

Levels of training: Training is obviously the most straightforward way of equipping teachers with the knowledge to teach about HIV. Over half of the Kenyan teachers reported not having received any training on HIV/AIDS. This figure is likely to be lower nationally because Nyanza has been the focus of an intensive teacher training programme on HIV. Training on HIV/AIDS in India appears to be even less common – 70 per cent of teachers said they had never received any training on HIV.

It takes special skills to talk about sex and a life-threatening disease, especially in countries where sex, and consequently HIV, are linked to immorality. These are big obstacles, but they can be overcome. However, these are not talents one can gain from a book: it will take a very different type of training and learning process to gain the necessary skills. More than anything, it is about communication.

Over-burdened timetable: Linked to the issue of staff shortages, teachers were asked whether or not they had enough time to teach HIV/AIDS: 52 per cent of Indian teachers and 55 per cent of Kenyan teachers said they did not.

In many countries there needs to be a fundamental review of the school curriculum to determine which topics are fundamental and relevant to school education. In many cases the national curriculum is already over-burdened, with new subjects or curriculum areas frequently added without anything ever being taken away. Over the years this has led to saturation—there simply isn't the space or the time for yet another new curriculum area on HIV/AIDS. It can exist on paper in Ministry of Education documents, but it will not appear in practice. Only by doing a more fundamental review of the entire curriculum can new space be found which will make it possible for HIV/AIDS education to be seriously addressed.

Gender: A recurring theme in the interviews was the reported shyness felt by teachers in talking about HIV/AIDS with members of the opposite sex. This gender dimension appeared to be stronger in India then Kenya.

The gender issue has two implications for teaching HIV/AIDS. If possible, training should be designed to overcome inhibitions that teachers have in discussing sex with students of the opposite gender. Alternatively, if inhibitions about having a frank discussion about sex with the opposite gender are too ingrained, then there is merit in having single sex lessons.

Role models: There has been concern that teachers do not act as positive role models for young people, and that their own sexual behaviour is in direct contradiction to the behaviour they advocate in HIV/AIDS education. In order to investigate this claim, all respondents were asked that whether, on the whole, teachers in their school set a good example to pupils when it came to safe sexual behaviour.

In Kenya, 23 per cent of students said that teachers did not set a good example with regards to sexual behaviour. A much smaller percentage (9 per cent) of teachers reported the same. Among parents the figure was 17 per cent. In India, teachers were regarded as better role models for sexual behaviour than in Kenya, with 13 per cent of students, 4 per cent of teachers and only 3 per cent of parents saying they thought teachers did not set a good example.

Some of the interviews in Kenya indicated that teacher-pupil sexual relationships were occurring. For teachers to have sexual relationships with students is both illegal and a gross infringement of the power a teacher holds over a student. The education and legal systems have the responsibility to ensure that teachers who are found to be having sexual relations with students are prosecuted.

Key Recommendations

a) Myths and misconceptions about HIV are potentially very harmful and need to be challenged in schools. Teachers must be able to explain clearly to young people why they are false.

b) There is a need to have public fora discussing HIV/AIDS and the role the school plays in educating young people about HIV and sex. Communication between parents and educational personnel will mean that parental expectations of the school will match the teachers' perceived responsibilities.

c) Ownership of the curriculum must be broadened to involve parents, teachers and religious leaders as stakeholders. However, these stakeholders must first go through an educational process themselves in which they can begin to discuss sensitive issues such as sexual and gender relations. During this process, they will be able to identify the positive role they can play in HIV/AIDS education, and start to take responsibility for it.

d) Taking advantage of pre-existing systems of knowledge transfer—mothers, peers and, where appropriate, the extended family system should be targeted and encouraged to communicate on HIV/AIDS in positive, open and accurate ways.

e) To ensure clear and consistent messages, HIV/AIDS education must target all sectors of society including religious leaders, the media, and families. It must look to provide the necessary knowledge about HIV, and learning must be participatory and locally relevant.

f) Learning resources on HIV/AIDS should be locally driven, drawing upon local statistics of prevalence and case studies. This will make it easier for students to view HIV as a problem which is relevant to their own lives – an issue which can affect 'us', not just 'them'. Close links must also be made with other agencies collecting and collating local data – to ensure it can inform discussions in local schools.

g) HIV/AIDS education needs to draw upon a wide range of creative pedagogic tools and in doing so can contribute to wider change in schools. Rote learning or learning passively from textbooks is not a useful approach when it comes to HIV/AIDS. In order to really engage children and change their attitudes or behaviour a different model of learning is needed. The use of song, dance, visualisation, story telling, role play and drama are just a few of the approaches that can help children to connect more deeply.

h) Governments should encourage the development of mobile external resource teams within every district. External resource teams have the advantage of being able to more easily raise sensitive issues such as sex and HIV. Teachers will then be in a better position to follow up on these issues as there will be a precedent of openess. If such groups are promoted, not just at a national level, but also at a district level, then they can realistically reach all schools and can also contribute to wider education for parents, religious leaders, etc.

REFERENCES

Barnett E., De Koning K. and Francis V., "Health and HIV/AIDS Education in primary and secondary schools in Africa and Asia", *Education Research*, London, Department for International Development, 1995.

Barnett T. and Whiteside A., *AIDS in the Twenty–First Century*, Chippenham and Eastbourne, Antony Rowe Ltd., 2002.

Bundy D., *Education and HIV/AIDS: A Window of Hope*, Washington DC, The World Bank, 2002.

Coombe, C., , Kelly M., "Education as a vehicle for combating HIV/AIDS", *UNESCO Prospects*; 31(3): 435–445), 2001.

Kelly M., *Planning for Education in the context of HIV/AIDS*, Paris, IIEP, UNESCO, 2000.

Robert Holloway, "Lack of Awareness Hurts AIDS Prevention in Japan," *The Daily Yomiuri*, August 11, 1990.

Ronald Bayer, *Private Acts, Social Consequences: AIDS and the Politics of Public Health,* New Brunswick, M. J.: Rutgers University Press, 1991.

World Health Organisation (WHO), *AIDS: Global Situation*, New Delhi, India: Southeast Asia Regional Office, 1992.

3

Guidance and Counselling of HIV/AIDS

HIV counselling is a confidential dialogue between a client and a counsellor aimed at enabling the client to cope with stress and take personal decisions related to HIV/AIDS. The counselling process includes evaluating the personal risk of HIV transmission, and discussing how to prevent infection. It concentrates specifically one motional and social issues related to possible or actual infection with HIV and to AIDS. With the consent of the client, counselling can be extended to spouses, sex partners and relatives.

HIV counselling has as its objectives both prevention and care. A counsellor is a person trained in the skills of the job: listening to the client, asking supportive questions, discussing options, encouraging the client to make his or her own informed decisions, giving practical information and suggesting follow-up. Counselling should be a process involving a series of sessions as well as follow-up. It can bed one in any location that offer peace of mind and confidentiality for the client.

Two types of counselling, according to site, are practised. Clinic-based counselling is counselling provided in a formal session-in a hospital, health centre or clinic-by a trained professional, such as a doctor, social worker, nurse or psychologist. Community-based counselling is given in a non-formal environment, in a village or urban neighbourhood-by one community member trained in counselling to another community or family member.

PRE-TEST COUNSELLING

HIV counselling is often given in connection with a voluntary HIV test. Such counselling helps to prepare the client for the HIV test, explains the implications of knowing that one is or is not infected with HIV, and facilitates discussion about ways to cope with knowing one's HIV status. It also involves a discussion of sexuality, relationships, possible sex- and drug-related risk behaviours, and how to prevent infection. It helps correct myths and misinformation around the subject of AIDS. Whenever resources permit, pre-test counselling should be made available to those who desire it. People who do not want or do not have access to pre-test counselling should not be prevented from taking a voluntary HIV test, however. In contrast, informed consent is always required before an HIV test where the individual's name will be linked to the result.

POST-TEST COUNSELLING

Post-test counselling helps the client understand and cope with the HIV test result. Here, the counsellor prepares the client for the result, gives the result and then provides the client with any further information required, if necessary referring the person to other services. The two usually discuss ways to reduce the risk of infection or transmission. HIV test results should always be given with counselling. The form of post-test counselling will depend on what the test result is. Where it is positive, the counsellor needs to tell the client clearly, and as gently and humanly as possible, providing emotional support and discussing with the client on how best to cope, including information on relevant referral services.

Ongoing counselling will help clients accept their HIV status, and take a positive attitude to their lives. Through ongoing counselling the infected person may choose to invite a trusted family member to share confidentiality and participate in the counselling-enabling the family to start practising family level counselling.

Counselling is also important after a negative result. While the client is likely to feel relief, the counsellor must emphasise several points. First, because of the "window period", a negative result may not mean absence of infection, and the client might wish to consider returning fora repeat test after three-six months. Second, counsellors need to discuss HIV prevention, providing support to help the client adopt and sustain any new safer practices.

COUNSELLING FOR BEHAVIOURAL CHANGE

The availability of HIV counselling, even without HIV testing, may create a private environment for discussing sexual matters and personal worries. Counselling augments AIDS education by making HIV related information personally relevant. Counselling of this type for behavioural change has been successfully provided in the Medical Research Council project in western Uganda. Here, community-based counselling in a small rural community increased condom use from 2,000 to 7,000 per month.

COUNSELLING FOR CHILDREN

In many places, children are increasingly affected by the epidemic. Apart from those themselves infected with HIV, they include children where one or both of the parents are either living with HIV or AIDS or have died of AIDS. These children have special counselling needs, such as the emotional trauma of seeing their parents being ill or die, discrimination by other children and adults, and emotional worries about their own continuing illness. Older children may need counselling related to sexual issues, and on the avoidance of risk behaviour.

COUNSELLING FOR PREGNANT WOMEN

Counselling can benefit pregnant women—or women wanting to become pregnant—who are either HIV-positive or unaware of their HIV status. It facilitates their making informed decisions about whether to become pregnant Counselling and HIV/AIDS: UNAIDS Technical Update if HIV-infected; whether to take a test before pregnancy; and, if pregnant, whether to terminate the pregnancy, where abortion is legally available.

For those already pregnant, counselling can also discuss the use of zidovudine (ZDV, also known as AZT), where available, to reduce the risk of transmitting HIV to the unborn child, and breast-feeding and other infant feeding options. Where possible, and when the woman agrees, it is advantageous to involve her male partner in the counselling sessions. Ideally, women should have counselling available to them before they become pregnant.

COUPLE COUNSELLING

This is sometimes provided to a pair of sex partners, who agree to attend sessions together. It can help resolve misunderstandings between the two people—such as over worries when one of them is tested HIV-positive—that can lead in some cases to violence, particularly against women. Couple counselling can also be given to a client and his or her sex partner or spouse, before or after an HIV test. It is also provided as part of premarital counselling.

OBSTACLES OF HIV COUNSELLING

Various obstacles stand in the way of HIV counselling being provided effectively wherever necessary. An underlying problem is the fact that counselling may not be given its proper due by policymakers and service managers—in part, because of the inherent difficulty of measuring its quality and impact on psychological stress reduction and behaviour change. Because of this, priority is often not given to the proper planning of counselling services and counsellors may not receive the official approval and resources they need to do their job effectively. Another major constraint is the lack of good counselling training schedules that are applicable to local circumstances.

Poor Selection of Trainees for Counselling

People are sometimes put on training courses simply because they are "due" for another course, or to fill up the course, and not because they will be taking up positions as counsellors. This is one reason why those trained in counselling often do not continue to practise it.

Lack of Supervised Practice and Follow-up after Training

Since counselling is a skill dependent on the personal qualities of warmth and understanding, it is often mistakenly assumed to require little in the way of preparation and practical training. For this reason, a two-three-day workshop, without any supervised practice, is sometimes felt to be enough to produce a trained counsellor.

Inadequate Resources, Facilities and Organisation

Problems frequently encountered relating to poor organisation or insufficient resources include the following.

a) Counselling is not considered an essential social service, and there are therefore no clear policies on funding.

b) There is a lack of confidentiality.

c) The setting of the service is inappropriate for clients because of lack of privacy during counselling sessions, inconvenient opening times or difficult physical access.

d) The procedure of the service is intimidating, for example, clients may be interrogated by reception staff.

e) Counsellors often have an established job-such as nursing-which is regarded as taking priority over counselling. Without priority or proper resources being given to counselling, many counsellors have to carry out home visits in their spare time, as a voluntary activity. The consequent frustration can result in burnout.

f) Clients are not referred at the right time. For example, clients may not have been offered pre-test counselling-or possibly have not even given informed consent to testing-and may come to the counsellor, panic-stricken, on learning they are HIV-positive, the counsellor is then required to sort this situation out. If this happens repeatedly in spite of the counsellor's complaints it may burn out the ability to cope.

Often, counsellors are able to provide only a single post-test counselling session and do not make follow-up plans because they are overwhelmed with other duties, or because they lack transport for home visits.

Burnout

Burnout is a state of emotional exhaustion, that results when the counsellor has reached his or her limit to deal with HIV and the emotional stress it causes. This may lead to a state of irritability and anger, often directed at supervisors, colleagues and even clients. The counsellor may also feel despair at the limited number of sources of social or medical support that can be suggested to the client, especially in communities starved of resources. The counsellor may have a privileged awareness of issues directly affecting the client's ability to cope and reduce future risk behaviour, and feel responsible for the client's welfare. However, because of lack of formal recognition and resources, counsellors may find they have few options to assist the client.

IMPORTANCE OF HIV COUNSELLING

One way counselling can be accorded its proper respect is by conducting studies on its delivery, quality and impact. Research findings on counselling can help convince decision makers and service managers to endorse and provide resources in support of counselling services. In Uganda, TASO (The AIDS Service Organisation) conducted a study on 730 HIV-positive clients to whom it had given long-term counselling. Counselling appeared to help these clients cope with their infection. Of the clients sampled, 90 per cent had revealed the fact of their infection to another person, with 85.3 per cent telling relations. The study also showed a high level of acceptance of HIV-positive people with in families (79 per cent) and in communities (76 per cent), as reported by the TASO clients who had received regular counselling. After results were discussed at each hospital where TASO operated, the hospital managers provided more space for counsellors and encouraged doctors to refer clients to TASO counsellors.

In 1992, a study in Rwanda examined the impact of preventive counselling. It was shown that for the women whose partners were also tested and counselled, the annual incidence of new HIV infections decreased from 4.1 per cent to 1.8 per cent. Among women who were HIV positive, the prevalence of gonorrhoea decreased from 13 per cent to 6 per cent, with the greatest reduction in those using condoms. As a result of these findings, counselling was recognised as a mainstream intervention and the funders of the study established a project for counselling and discordant couples in Zambia.

Proper Selection of Trainees for Counselling

Candidates for a counselling training course should satisfy a number of conditions. They must be given a job description that specifies that they can provide counselling. They must have the necessary agreed professional background—this may be as a social worker, health worker, teacher, community worker, or a volunteer from a group of people living with HIV/AIDS. They should be good listeners, respected by others, motivated and resilient, and have warm and caring personalities.

In order to select people with good qualities for counselling, TASO uses the following approach. First, prospective trainees must have a job placement where they can see clients who require counselling. Second, TASO conducts a one day AIDS counselling awareness workshop for a large group of people being considered for training. This awareness workshop must be conducted separately from training on the technical skills of counselling.

During the awareness workshop, a number of issues concerning AIDS—including controversial matters such as compulsory partner notification—are brought up. The trainers observe the attitudes, reactions and interpersonal interaction skills of the prospective trainees, and based on this, select people for the actual skills training. In order to chose the right type of people to become counsellors, those selecting trainees should have a good understanding of the cultural context in which counselling is to be delivered.

Training Workshop, followed by Supervised Practice

Most of the current effort in training takes the form of a single workshop, with no follow-up supervision. Instead, after the initial workshop the trained person should be placed in counselling work, with support and good supervision, and should participate in a second training workshop later.

Such an approach has been followed in several places. The Zambian national AIDS programme, for instance, has set up a countrywide programme for training in HIV counselling. This begins with a basic workshop, followed by placement in a work situation, which is later followed up by an advanced workshop.

Retention of Trained Counsellors

In Tanzania, a study showed that of those who had received counselling training, less than a quarter were reported to be practising counselling. Counsellors often leave their jobs, most probably because of burnout and lack of proper support. If counsellors are given proper support, the stresses which can build up and cause burn out can be reduced. Such support can take three forms:

a) administrative support, including the provision of better working facilities and timetables, and job descriptions that accommodate counselling;
b) professional support, where a supervisor discusses cases with the counsellor or provides emotional support;
c) peer support from colleagues.

Service Development and Support

Once the heads of service sites and AIDS programmes are convinced of the importance of counselling, then one can get down to establishing the basics for a good service.

Excessive workloads on counsellors that lead to burnout can be reduced by using trained part-time volunteers and a well planned system of shifts, for example, a nurse may do counselling for four hours in the morning, and then work at the nurse station in the afternoon.

a) The location and opening hours of the service should take into account the needs of the particular community. Counselling has been carried out in STD clinics, hospital outpatient departments and hospital wards. Some non-governmental organisations (NGOs) have set-up counselling centres inside hospital compounds. Others have established counselling services on their own premises, or in centres specially dedicated to HIV counselling. Counselling services for sex workers, as well as condom supplies, are sometimes offered in the vicinity of night clubs, and operate at night.
b) HIV/AIDS educational campaigns should include details on how, where and when people can obtain counselling.
c) Reception staff should be trained to adopt a supportive and sympathetic attitude, and sensitised to the need for confidentiality.

d) If resources permit, counselling services for asymptomatic individuals, as well as preventive counselling, should be located separately from care services for AIDS patients. This enables those living with HIV but who have not yet developed AIDS to receive counselling without being depressed by seeing very ill AIDS patients.

e) Counselling sessions need to be well planned so that, for instance, informed consent is always sought and counselling offered before a client takes an HIV test.

f) Counselling should be integrated into other services, including STD, antenatal and family planning clinics.

g) Community-based counselling services can be initiated and expanded quickly and at little expense.

Referral Systems

The existence of good support for counsellors is directly related to the existence of a good referral system. A referral system should be developed in consultation with NGOs, community-based organisations, hospital directors and other service managers, as well as with networks of people living with HIV and AIDS. An efficient referral system will enable AIDS service organisations and other NGOs to refer clients requiring medical care to hospitals and clinics. At the same time medical services should refer clients to specialised NGOs for ongoing counselling, home care and social support, such as the provision of food and housing. In Abidjan, Côte d'Ivoire, NGOs such as Espoir work closely with Treichville University Hospital to provide medical, nursing and psychosocial care to inpatients and outpatients with HIV/AIDS. Espoir also operates a free, anonymous HIV counselling and testing centre.

At the Thai Red Cross Society, clients of the Anonymous Counselling Center are referred to the Wednesday Friends' Club (a support group for people living with HIV and AIDS) and the Chulalongkorn Hospital Immune Clinic for follow-upon treatment and care. Referrals should always be confidential, and clients should be advised to contact named individuals at the referral site, rather than being given a general referral note. A referral system can only function well if the referring care giver discusses with the client the reasons why he or she is being referred and the services which are available at the referral site. It is suggested that regular meetings should be held among service providers to review and improve the referral system.

HIV TESTING AND COUNSELLING SERVICES

HIV testing and counselling includes the HIV testing and counselling processes in clinical and preventive settings based on pre-test education and employing opt-out approaches to the increasingly routine offer of HIV testing. They are a gateway to entry points for HIV prevention, care and impact mitigation. Scaling up these services is a critical step for scaling up a range of HIV/AIDS prevention, care, treatment and support interventions. With increasing access to ARV treatment, the demand for HIV testing and counselling is likely to increase dramatically. Thus, there is an urgent need to scale up HIV testing and counselling services.

A public health approach for scaling up HIV testing and counselling services is based on the following guiding principles:

i) Building and sustaining political commitment for scaling up HIV testing and counselling in the context of HIV prevention, care, treatment and support is critical for working towards universal access to HIV testing and counselling.
ii) Quality HIV testing and counselling services must involve developing and supporting efforts to improve the awareness of the benefits of HIV testing and counselling. This will also help to normalise HIV and testing and counselling services. It will also help to reduce stigma and discrimination.

iii) Involving people with HIV, communities and other key stakeholders in planning, implementing, monitoring and evaluating HIV testing and counselling services is critical for ensuring appropriate and effective services and achieving good prevention and care outcomes.

iv) Developing and using standardised HIV testing and counselling protocols, as a part of a public health approach for scaling up testing and counselling, will be important for ensuring quality of services.

v) HIV testing and counselling services must be client-centred and have effective links to post-test services and support. Client-centred HIV testing and counselling services respond to the needs of clients and make the client feel accepted and valued.

vi) HIV testing and counselling services must be ethically appropriate. Mandatory HIV testing is not effective for public health purposes nor is it ethical. The following principles must be respected:

   a) HIV testing must be voluntary.

   b) Confidentiality must be protected.

   c) Accountability.

Policy Development

Policy development for counselling and testing services must be addressed at operational, national and international levels. Policy is a tool that provides adequate framework and support at every level. While national and international policy frameworks and advocacy—a process to bring about change in laws, policies and practices, are an essential background to counselling and testing services at the national level, it is also clear that policy and advocacy have an equal and complementary role at local, implementation level. They can be used to engage stakeholders and resources, to challenge legal frameworks, address issues of equity and social justice, and to harmonise services within specific areas. Policy and advocacy are necessary as for creating and maintaining motivation and support for quality in service delivery, for example through accreditation or validation processes.

An enabling policy environment is one that comprehensively addresses political, economic, social, legal and health issues so that people will not feel discouraged about learning their status. Such issues form the environment which efforts to combat HIV/AIDS take place. The ways in which these issues are engaged can either enable or disable HIV testing and counselling services to a marked degree. The development of enabling policies aims to guide and support implementation of HIV testing and counselling services.

Building Political Commitment

Endorsement, active involvement and leadership by people in positions of authority is vital for implementing HIV testing and counselling services and care, treatment and prevention programmes, as well as for combating stigma and discrimination. This is 'political' in its broadest sense — it means involving those who have influence and decision-making capacity that affects the lives of those affected by HIV, not only in the areas of health and social welfare, but also in aspects of business, law, politics and economics. These people are most often the 'gatekeepers' who can allow or block, intentionally or not, many aspects of tackling the HIV epidemic. Once gatekeepers have been identified, strategic information can be shared with them and other partners can be mobilised.

Political commitment to mobilising resources is critical to the successful planning and implementation of counselling and testing services. Resource mobilisation will mean identifying possible sources and opportunities, setting clear priorities, demonstrating success, sharing strategic information and building capacity for resource mobilisation.

Involving Stakeholders

Since HIV is not just a health problem but also a social, political, legal and economic one, one cannot over-stress the importance of involving and mobilising a range of stakeholders in dealing with the epidemic, both because they are affected and because they can play a number of different roles. Involving and mobilising a range of stakeholders means making serious efforts to build and maintain relationships within and across different sectors of society—formal and informal, within government, community, business and civil society. It should happen at all levels, i.e, central and implementation levels and should be coordinated. While each stakeholder will have his or her own reasons for entering into partnership or collaboration over counselling and testing services, it is important to keep differing interests balanced and focused on the primary purpose which is the support of people with HIV and promotion of public health.

Involving Public

Ensuring the greater and more meaningful involvement of people with HIV in all aspects of HIV testing and counselling services is a true reflection of political commitment. Too often this has remained a principle and has not been translated into action.

The greater and more meaningful involvement of people with HIV in all aspects of HIV testing and counselling services is also consistent with a rights-based approach, which acknowledges that people have a part to play in decisions that affect their lives. Supporting people to play an effective part in decisions that affect their lives is critical for ensuring greater involvement. This applies as much to HIV testing and counselling as to any other area of policy or action.

Promoting a Rights-based Approach

Promoting a right based approach to HIV testing and counselling services will help to normalise HIV testing and counselling in health facilities and in communities. It is also critical for improving people's perceptions about the benefits of HIV testing and counselling and this has a direct impact on the uptake of services.

Most countries are signatories to international legal instruments, declarations and guidelines that are critical components of the rights-based approach to HIV testing and counselling services. Being a signatory to these instruments creates an obligation for signatory countries to adhere to the principles laid down in the instruments, under public international law. The instruments form a framework of rights that gives states a basis to formulate their local laws, policies and practices. International instruments provide standards that facilitate the creation of an enabling environment for HIV testing and counselling.

The most significant barriers that deny people access to HIV testing and counselling are stigmatising laws and practices. These discriminate against vulnerable populations such as sex workers, injecting drug users, men who have sex with men, women and children, and include laws that discriminate against people with HIV on issues of employment, marriage and founding a family, and denial of access to health care and medicines.

Persistent stigma and discrimination prevent people from seeking HIV testing and counselling. Stigmatising, discriminatory laws impede public health objectives and should be repealed or reformed. There must be careful attention to ensure that such vulnerable populations have access to ethical, appropriate and effective HIV testing and counselling services, otherwise the existing inequities and inequalities will only be exacerbated.

The regulatory environment affecting medicines and medical supplies, including laboratory and prevention commodities A complex regulatory environment affects medicines and essential commodities including laboratory and prevention supplies. It requires close attention to detail in order to ensure that the supply chain can deliver the materials necessary for providing HIV testing and counselling services. It concerns regulation of the quality and safety of medicines and medical supplies, of who may use them, the regulation of trade, the use of public money for medical supplies, and sanctions for misuse or misappropriation.

The regulatory environment for medicines and medical supplies will involve cooperation and collaboration between ministries of health, trade, finance and home affairs. It will cover transactions within particular countries but also extends to goods sourced from outside the country. The question of intellectual property rights is important in the use and availability of medicines and other technologies, but other trade considerations must also be taken into account, for example import licensing and taxation of imports and sales of medicines and other goods. Legislation and other measures to protect valuable commodities from theft must also be considered, since they will be particularly vulnerable in conditions of scarcity, when they have high value for illegal trading.

Health Sector Policies

Health sector policies may be enshrined within national legislation on health or HIV/AIDS and regulations may be in place to enforce these policies. Once again, it is important to assess health sector policies as part of the process of planning and implementing HIV testing and counselling services. They include:

i) HIV prevention and care policies, which are likely to include, HIV testing and counselling, prevention mother-to-child HIV transmission (PMTCT), post-exposure prophylaxis (PEP) for health and emergency workers or for sexual assault victims, universal precautions (UP) to prevent unintended transmission of HIV, TB prevention and treatment and ARV treatment.

ii) Public health approaches to HIV/AIDS, including provision of HIV testing and counselling. These should address questions such as who may conduct an HIV test and how HIV testing and counselling may be supported to achieve the best public health benefit. Leveraging of human resources must be addressed to deal with increasing numbers of people seeking HIV testing and counselling, including financing, recruitment, training, quality assurance and accreditation of facilities and health care workers.

Quality and safety of medicines and medical supplies for use in HIV testing and counselling programmes is the responsibility of the Health Ministry's Drug Regulatory Authority (DRA) and other bodies responsible for regulation medical supplies. Regulations of these bodies will indicate the conditions under which new supplies may be registered, and who is allowed to dispense or sell these commodities.

Regulations for the selection and use of medicines and medical supplies including laboratory and prevention commodities may exist at national level, or may be developed for local use in accordance with any existing regulations, determining HIV testing strategies, protocols for HIV testing and counselling in different health care settings.

Funding mechanisms for medicines and medical supplies including laboratory and prevention commodities — how HIV testing and counselling services will be funded, and how the public or programme users will be expected to contribute towards costs through cost-sharing mechanisms, subsidies service fees or other models.

Community Mobilisation

When planning and implementing HIV testing and counselling services, it is essential to also plan and implement community mobilisation activities. Social mobilisation for HIV testing and counselling means to provide the community with adequate information and support about all aspects of the counselling and testing services. This enables:

i) community members to make informed decisions about HIV testing and counselling
ii) normalisation of HIV testing and counselling services and knowing one's status
iii) acceptance of HIV/AIDS as an important issue for the community
iv) community involvement and participation in HIV testing and counselling services
v) increased uptake of counselling and testing services
vi) reduction of denial, stigma and discrimination.

Encouraging community members to talk about counselling and HIV testing is a very important part of community action on HIV/AIDS. Talking about HIV testing and counselling can raise very personal issues about people's private lives. Encouraging communities to talk about HIV testing and counselling must be handled with sensitivity and respect. It is important for those working with communities to understand the facts and issues around HIV testing and counselling before they encourage community members to talk about these issues and to become involved in HIV testing and counselling. Increasing the acceptance of HIV as a community issue also mobilises community members to respond to HIV/AIDS. Increasingly, community mobilisation in of itself is being seen as an important HIV/AIDS intervention.

Increasing demand for HIV testing and counselling services is critical for normalising HIV, increasing acceptance of HIV as a community issue and reducing denial, stigma and discrimination. However, because of the stigma and discrimination that is associated with HIV/AIDS, many people are afraid of knowing their status. Community mobilisation for HIV testing and counselling must therefore address stigma and discrimination, fear of disclosure as well as people's perceptions of the benefits of HIV testing and counselling. In some settings, mass media and marketing approaches have proven quite successful in improving people's perceptions about the benefits of knowing one's status and increasing uptake of HIV testing and counselling.

Comomodity Management

Reliable and affordable supplies of commodities are critical for success of HIV testing and counselling services. Not only do they affect the quality of services, their availability and cost also affect uptake of HIV testing. An effective commodity management system must be in place to ensure their accessibility and effective use, both at service delivery level and in referral services. Commodity management for HIV testing and counselling services will follow well-established principles, but must be flexible and responsive to the varied settings and services offered.

Commodities for HIV testing and counselling services may include:

i) Laboratory tables/work benches
ii) HIV test kits
iii) Automated analysers, such as ELISA readers
iv) Reagents and controls
v) Centrifuges
vi) Refrigerators
vii) Test tubes, racks, timers, pipettes and other lab consumables
viii) Commodities for specimen collection–lancets, needles, syringes, plasters
ix) Commodities for universal precautions– disposable gloves, bleach, cleaning supplies, sharps disposal for needles and lancets, waste disposal bags for blood-contaminated materials

x) Male and female condoms and water-based lubricants

xi) Safe drinking water and cups

xii) Information materials for training and education

xiii) Equipment for providing training – TV, videos, flip charts, pens.

Managing drugs, diagnostic test kits and other health commodities in any setting (public or private sector) and at any level (local, regional or national) follows a well-recognised cycle of selection, procurement, distribution and use. Management support is at the centre of the cycle—its functions hold the cycle together. The entire cycle rests on a policy and legal framework that establishes the mechanisms for each function and supports the commodity management system.

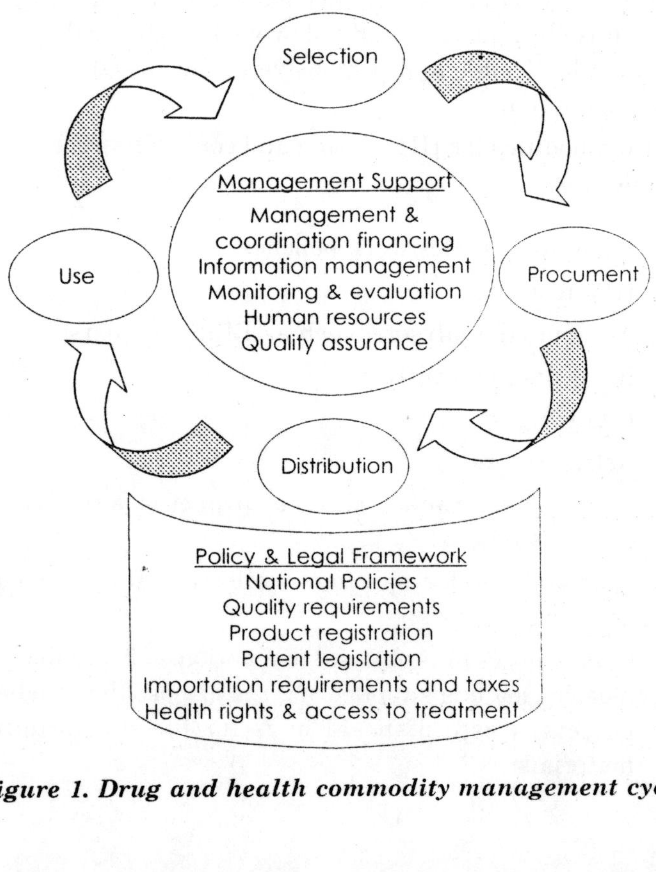

Figure 1. Drug and health commodity management cycle

Management Support

The essential functions of management support for HIV testing and counselling services includes:

i) *Financing:* lack of sufficient and continuous financing and failures in accounting systems for testing and counselling commodities have been widely reported, with consequent lack of HIV testing capacity and failure in support for prevention through condom supply;

ii) *Management and co-ordination:* Continuity of supply for HIV testing and counselling is essential to keep programmes functioning; at the same time, when large amounts of drugs and commodities are being procured and distributed, corruption and theft can become significant problems. Active and transparent management are essential throughout the system, with coordination between those responsible for every stage of the cycle, to minimise losses and maximise the services that can be provided with limited resources.

iii) *Quality assurance:* Commodity quality includes selection of products on the basis of safety and efficacy, ensuring good manufacturing practices are followed, ensuring suppliers can be trusted on product quality and on their delivery performance, protecting the quality of products during storage and transportation, removal of defective products and redistribution of overstocked products to ensure that they are used before expiry.

iv) *Information management, monitoring and evaluation:* These are crucial for good management

Policy and Legal Framework

It is important to be familiar with policies and legislation relevant to medical commodities for HIV testing and counselling services; these include:

i) National policies, such as the HIV testing policy, essential medicines policy and policies governing laboratory and medical practice.
ii) Quality requirements for tests, medicines, and good laboratory, distribution/storage, prescribing and dispensing practices.
iii) Product registration, which many countries enforce for medical commodities.
iv) Patent legislation, which affects what products are allowed to be traded and supplied in individual countries.
v) Importation requirements and taxes, which control entry of products into individual countries and can have a significant effect on costs through importation and sales taxes.

Policy decisions at service delivery level are also important for commodity management, including decisions on which services to provide, whether to use EIAs or rapid tests, whether to perform serial or parallel HIV testing, and whether to provide treatment services and for which health problems.

The national AIDS reference laboratory is responsible in many countries for deciding on the validity of different types of tests for use within a country and thus shaping choices for product selection, developing standard guidelines for product use and setting standards and procedures for monitoring product quality. The national medicines regulatory authority will provide similar support concerning any medicines or medical supplies that are used in testing and counselling services and can provide valuable advice on product sources, quality, patent status and safety for use in people with HIV.

Existing national or other bulk medical commodity procurement and distribution systems should be used wherever possible for setting up and maintaining the supply chain for testing and counselling services. These may be part of the national public health system or may be run independently by NGOs (especially faith-based health providers) or as cooperative buyers clubs (separate organisations working together to gain price advantages and coordinate distribution). It may be necessary to adapt strengthen such systems in order to cope with the added requirements of HIV testing and counselling services. If such adaptation and use of existing systems is not feasible, it will be necessary to set up a separate system, especially in the early stages. However, this should not be a long-term policy, since medical commodity procurement, especially for HIV-related services, is rapidly developing and requires considerable networking and market intelligence to make the best use of resources.

Commodity Selection

The first stage, before selection of commodities can begin, is to establish standard HIV testing algorithms/guidelines, and treatment guidelines for any related prevention, care or treatment services that require medicines. Development of guidelines requires expertise at national level, including clinical, financial and procurement input to ensure that guidelines are actually practicable in the various contexts within the country. The widespread application of such guidelines will help to make demand for commodities more predictable and easier to quantify. It will also ensure that product selection is based on expert consensus about which products are suitable and cost-effective for specific settings.

At national level:

a) national HIV testing guidelines or algorithms must be developed or regularly updated.
b) guidelines should include recommendations for procedures for HIV testing in smallscale settings as well as HIV testing in central or hospital laboratories.
c) guidelines must be available at testing and counselling facilities in both public and private sectors.
d) guidelines must be distributed to donors to ensure that any HIV test kit donations are compatible with national guidelines.

e) national standard treatment guidelines must be developed for prophylaxis and treatment of HIV-related diseases, and the required HIV-related medicines should be included in the national essential drugs list and/or formulary.

At service delivery level:

a) The national guidelines for testing and treatment should be used to identify which specific guidelines and algorithms are required for the interventions to be offered.
b) The specific guidelines should be checked for appropriateness to the local context of testing and counselling services and the available resources.
c) Other relevant guidelines should also be checked in the same way, such as those for TB, STIs, malaria and nutritional supplementation in HIV and/or pregnancy
d) If specific national guidelines are lacking or inappropriate for local use, local standard treatment guidelines must be developed.

Evaluation of HIV test kits should, preferably, be the responsibility of a national technical advisory group. In some countries, this group will be able to rely on a national central reference laboratory to evaluate accuracy and operational characteristics of the kits. This function might also be carried out by a regional laboratory or at a testing facility. The WHO pre-qualification scheme for HIV test kits can be relied upon for information about the different tests. Regional laboratories that are independent and non-commercial can be used to gain more information about use of tests in settings with similar epidemiological profiles. National evaluation is necessary to indicate which tests are appropriate for the population.

When standard guidelines have been developed and test kit evaluations have been examined, it is then possible to make selection of HIV test kits. Choices will depend on the following factors:

i) *Testing format:* Rapid tests which are based on enzyme immunoassays (EIAs) versus micro ELISA: this will depend on the volume of testing, local capacity and the importance of providing same-day results.

ii) *Sensitivity and specificity of tests:* The first test must have a sensitivity greater than 99 per cent, second and third tests must have a specificity greater than 99 per cent.

iii) *HIV variants and subgroups*: It is essential that the in-country evaluation ensures that the right tests are chosen for the HIV variants and subgroups present in the population.

iv) *Local capacity*: Selection of test kits must be appropriate for the language, training and experience of staff responsible for testing, and for the facilities available. Tests that require minimum equipment and handling of blood samples will help to reduce safety risks for staff, for example using whole blood finger prick samples rather than serum or plasma which must be centrifuged from samples drawn with needle and syringe.

v) *Packaging, shelf life and cost*: In low-volume settings, small pack sizes of single tests are less likely to remain unused by their expiry date; larger packs can be used in high-volume settings, depending on the shelf-life— since most HIV test kits have comparatively short shelf-lives, very little time might remain when they arrive in facilities at the end of a long supply chain.

vi) *Refrigeration and constant power supplies*: These are necessary to preserve the quality of some HIV test kits and reagents, but might not be available some or all of the time, especially in low-resource or remote settings.

Similar principles apply for other commodities—medicines, supplies and equipment. The National Drug (Medicines) Programme should be able to supply information on availability, quality and storage characteristics of medicines and some medical supplies. HIV-related and other national treatment guidelines will provide guidance which products are appropriate for different situations and conditions.

When selections have been made, a full list of all commodities must be drawn up so that implementation and procurement managers can take the next steps of quantification and procurement. The list will also make clear to service delivery personnel what products will be available to them for their work. The list must indicate if special storage conditions are required. It can also indicate which health care staff may use or prescribe which products. At service delivery level, the process of selection will require choices to be made from the national list of testing and counselling commodities, according to the service delivery model chosen and the range of services to be provided.

Commodity Procurement

Procurement of commodities follows several steps, including quantification, sourcing and pricing, and ensuring timely delivery to the central store.

Quantification: Deciding how much of each commodity to buy is the first practical step in procurement. Quantification depends on three possible sets of data:

i) *Past usage (consumption) within the programme, generally provided from wellmaintained stock records:* This is useful for well-established programmes with predictable needs but not for new or rapidly changing situations.

ii) *Usage in similar programmes or services, using records from those programmes or (sometimes) data from suppliers who are familiar with the programmes*: This is useful in new programmes or with new treatments, if the programmes or services are sufficiently similar for the comparison to be valid.

iii) *Patient morbidity data and standard treatment protocols, a combination of data which will reflect the actual context of a treatment programme if the figures are accurate*: This method is more time-consuming, but is useful in promoting the use of standard treatment and laboratory guidelines – but careful judgement is necessary when morbidity figures are likely to be inaccurate or areas of unmet need have not yet been assessed.

The principles for estimating quantity are the same at national and service delivery level. Quantification can only be done successfully if users follow agreed policies and guidelines and have based their selection of commodities on them. If not, usage patterns are likely to be erratic and it will be difficult or impossible to decide how much of each commodity should be procured. Accurate quantification is important for two key reasons:

i) Ensuring that sufficient of each product is purchased, with adequate expiry dates, to ensure that there are no stock-outs and that each patient receives what they need, when they need it.
ii) Ensuring that not too much of each product is bought, resulting in wastage and overexpenditure due to products expiring on the shelf before they can be used.

Sourcing and pricing: It is important to establish good linkages with businesses involved in commodity supply, developing relationships that enable testing and counselling services to reach their goals. Good business relationships will provide motivation for suppliers to perform well, to avoid exploitation and to respond flexibly and helpfully to public health needs, especially during times of uncertainty. The process of sourcing and pricing of commodities involves:

i) Identifying who produces the required commodities and who will act as suppliers
ii) Verifying the quality of the producer and supplier as well of the products they offer, including the quality of service, continuity of production and ability to deliver on time.

iii) Identifying who can offer the best price when confidence has been established about the quality and equivalence of comparable versions of a particular product.

iv) Negotiating to obtain further price advantages on the basis of quantity and competition

Sourcing requires market intelligence, meaning active research of the global and local markets and of possibilities for procurement within and from outside a particular country. Commodities identified for procurement through the selection process may be:

i) *multiple-source (generic and innovator),* especially if a product is no longer controlled by patent regulations and competition exists between equivalent versions, for example drugs, dressings and condoms.

ii) *single-source (innovator)* if the patent-holder has a monopoly of the market for the product in a particular country; this applies to proprietary HIV tests and to new medicines.

iii) *single-source (generic or innovator)* if the product is off patent but not commercially profitable and only available from one producer.

Procurement officers might require external assistance in gathering information about sources, both within the country and from the international market. Information can be obtained for HIV-related single-source (innovator) commodities, or about both generic and innovator products through UN agencies and a number of international NGOs. WHO and NGOs such as Medecins sans Frontieres (MSF) and Health Action International (HAI) have produced a number of helpful documents on various aspects of sources, prices and patents, which are regularly updated and can be accessed via the internet.

Other important considerations in deciding on sources and acceptable prices include the delivery periods that suppliers can offer and their reliability in practice. Unreliable deliveries can be seriously harmful for individuals, programme success and credibility, so ability to achieve timely delivery must be considered as well as quality and price. Requirements for storage space must also be considered during the process of supplier selection and price negotiation, both for individual products and for bulk supplies.

Individual products may have special temperature requirements for storage, which will affect provision of facilities during procurement and after dispensing to the patient, especially in hot or extremely cold countries. The bulk volume of supplies depends on the packaging as well as on the product, and different suppliers may provide equivalent products in vastly different volumes; assessment must therefore be made of dimensions and storage requirements before placing a firm order for a product.

Donations might be considered or suggested as a source of HIV tests and medicines for under-funded programmes. However, experience shows that there are severe constraints to their usefulness for ongoing public health programmes. There are often significant hidden costs for 'free' gifts, including registration fees, customs duties, storage and distribution costs. Donors are often unable to supply tests and medicines that conform exactly to those listed in national or local guidelines.

Continuity of supply usually cannot be guaranteed over a prolonged period, which would affect the continuity and quality of testing services. An added constraint is that many rapid HIV tests have a short shelf life from the date of production. Recipients might easily find themselves with the problem of destroying unwanted or expired test kits in situations with very limited waste disposal facilities. However, there has been some success with carefully planned and controlled single source donation schemes, for example ivermectin for river blindness and nevirapine for PMTCT. The Interagency Guidelines for

Drug Donations should be followed on this subject and WHO/ EDM should be consulted for advice on the ways in which donation programmes can be implemented and made successful.

Pricing is usually done at the same time as sourcing and is the responsibility of procurement staff. Several lists of indicative prices exist for HIV-related commodities, which can be used for the selection process and at the beginning of price negotiations. A supplier might offer individual products from a standard price list, but there are often possibilities for downward negotiation of prices, especially for bulk purchases or regular repeat orders.

Individual programmes or facilities may not be able to achieve sufficient order volume to gain the best prices, but experience with procurement of essential drugs has shown that joint procurement arrangements between programmes or through a national clearing-house can allow for downward negotiation of prices. Examples include the Organisation of Eastern Caribbean States (OECS) Drug Procurement Service and church-related services such as MEDS in Kenya and Joint Medical Stores in Uganda. Some individual innovator companies have agreed to sell their products at significantly lower cost under price agreements for resource-limited countries experiencing serious public health problems; well-resourced countries will pay higher prices for the same products. Suppliers of differentially priced products generally seek safeguards to ensure that there is no 'leakage' of low-price products into countries that are not part of the price agreement. In other countries, the government sets maximum price levels or 'reference' prices that indicate the maximum that the public health system will pay for each product.

Quality Assurance

Quality must be the primary consideration in choosing what commodities to procure, especially for HIV tests and medicines. It must not be compromised by pricing or other considerations.

Quality assurance of medicines and health commodities ensures that products are consistently produced and monitored, so that patient safety is protected and testing or treatment interventions achieve reliable results and the maximum benefit. There must be proof that production facilities and procedures, distribution and storage conditions are of sufficient and consistent quality to provide confidence that the commodities will be safe and effective when used. Key activities for quality assurance quality include:

i) using recognised and trusted suppliers who supply good-quality products and backup services;
ii) pre-qualification of suppliers, especially for bulk procurement at national level, so that all concerned are aware of which products and suppliers have been approved;
iii) exchanging experiences between programmes and providers about quality of suppliers and products, at service delivery and procurement level, to build up knowledge and expertise for quality assurance.

Well-established guidelines on good manufacturing practice and quality assurance are provided by WHO and a number of internationally recognised regulatory authorities. Individual countries may also have such guidelines in place. Guidelines also exist for good storage, distribution and dispensing practice. Application of these guidelines will assist in providing good quality tests, medicines and supplies whose quality is maintained from the time of production until the commodities are put into use for the care of patients.

Monitoring of quality throughout the procurement system requires considerable technical expertise and facilities. These will be available in some countries, often administered by the Medicines Regulatory Authority. Regulatory systems are at different stages of development in different countries but are one of the chief means for a country to regulate what medicines are supplied to the public and to prevent substandard or ineffective medicines from being used. External assistance is available through WHO and other bodies when in-country capacity is lacking.

Pre-qualification of products and suppliers: The pre-qualification of suppliers and products is a process of verifying the manufacturer's claims about quality assurance, good Manufacturing practice and other standards, and verification of the quality and safety of commodities such as medicines and tests. Many countries and programmes lack adequate testing laboratories and the process of verifying supplier claims about quality is time-consuming and requires special expertise.

A number of schemes exist to share verified information about the quality of pharmaceuticals and of HIV tests. These schemes have focused on evaluating products and manufacturers of the new 'essential' commodities for treatment of HIV. The WHO schemes aim particularly at providing assistance for countries without local capacity for quality assurance or testing. The drugs pre-qualification list includes both generic and originator drugs.

When preparing to select the commodities to be used, independent information on the patent situation of medicines and tests should be sought. There are ongoing efforts by WHO, MSF and others to enable easier access to this information and quicker purchase of good quality drugs.

Reliance on the WHO lists of pre-qualified HIV diagnostics and medicines is strongly recommended. It saves time and effort, and provides independent verification of claims about quality. However, the fact that a product or producer is not listed does not necessarily mean that they are of bad quality—simply that they have not yet satisfied requirements for inclusion in the scheme. The pre-qualification list is constantly being revised and extended, so an uptodate version must always be consulted. In-country procurement managers can also set up their own pre-qualification schemes where facilities and human resources are adequate for this.

Procurement methods

Procurement methods vary according to product availability, quantity required and price. Procurement at a centralised national procurement facility will have the advantage of a concentration of skill, experience and bulk handling capacity. This is likely to be crucial when careful monitoring of supply and demand is required. Procurement might alternatively be decentralised to service provision level to allow greater control and responsiveness to change at local level.

Methods for procurement include:

i) competitive bidding or tendering (either open or limited),
ii) 'shopping' (comparison of quotations) for off-the-shelf small quantities
iii) contracting with specific suppliers for a period of repeat supply,
iv) procurement from UN or not-for-profit supply agencies.

Different methods will be required for different commodities and quantities. Some donors will impose their own guidelines for procurement when using their funds, for example, the World Bank. Procurement staff must understand the range of options and their advantages or disadvantages. In some instances, existing donor guidelines may introduce long delays before orders can be placed with suppliers. It may be necessary to negotiate with donors to streamline procedures so that HIV programmes are not held back from providing testing and treatment services.

Commodity Distribution

Careful management of distribution, including storage and transport, is essential for smooth running of the supply cycle and ensuring continuity of supply. This has four aims:

i) ensuring maintenance of product quality,
ii) reducing wastage

iii) preventing theft, pilfering or diversion to outlets other than the one intended

iv) controlling use and gathering information for ongoing procurement needs.

The processes of storage and distribution occur at several stages in the supply chain. They require adequate premises and transport facilities that are secure, of sufficient capacity for the volume of goods to be handled and maintained in a state designed to preserve the quality of the goods. This means that they must be clean and dry, with goods stored off the floor, adequate temperature control, and sufficient space between goods to facilitate handling and stock control. Different commodities require different storage and distribution conditions, particularly if they are temperature sensitive. These requirements must be included when assessing storage and distribution needs.

Inventory control: Inventory or stock control refers to the amount, location and value of each commodity within a supply system. Management of inventory depends on information systems that provide methods and feedback for:

a) tracking storage and movement of goods at every level within the supply system, from central storage through to stocks ready for use at the health facility;

b) ensuring proper stock rotation—it is essential to issue products with expiry dates such as HIV tests and medicines, so that items with the shortest expiry dates are used first

c) enabling managers to know the total amounts of a commodity that are within the supply system, and where, allowing redistribution or emergency supply when needed

d) recording acquisition and issue of stocks and

e) providing data for monitoring and further procurement.

Simple systems of inventory control can provide adequate data for most programmes and may be paper or computer based. Access to supplies must be restricted to those commodities that are permitted for use within the programme. Inventory records must be regularly monitored, to provide assurance that items are being issued correctly and not diverted or misused.

Good quality of inventory records is also essential to provide data for review and decisions about future procurement. In changeable conditions, such as the scaling up HIV testing and counselling services, it is essential to review inventory levels frequently, such as every month, rather than the six-monthly or annual review usually employed for inventory control. It is also important to remember to include within inventory sufficient stock for occasional unforeseen problems or emergencies.

Commodity Use

Use of commodities completes the supply management cycle, but is also the starting point of a new cycle of selection, procurement, distribution and use. Supply aspects that are important at the point where commodities are put into use include:

a) Adherence to guidelines for HIV testing, counselling, diagnosis or prevention
b) Recording which commodities are used for which patients and why
c) Feedback into the supply system of data required for planning continuity and further procurement, including prescribing, dispensing and laboratory records
d) Feedback about product acceptability to patients
e) Communicating requirements for new products or changes in guidelines which will result in variations in usage and changes in procurement

f) Stock management principles must be introduced at all levels

Prescribing and patient support: These are primarily clinical and technical responsibilities for technologists, doctors, nurses and pharmacists, but it is also essential that there are mechanisms for two-way exchange of information between clinical staff and procurement staff. Since continuity is critical in HIV prevention and care, it depends to a high degree on the continued efficiency and reliability of supply.

Monitoring and evaluation: Systems for monitoring and evaluation of the supply management cycle must include methods of matching data about performance of supply cycle with the experience at service delivery level. Methods exist for monitoring usage of essential medicines, which can be applied to HIV testing and counselling and treatment services. Methods also exist for monitoring effectiveness within procurement systems. However, there is little published information yet about methods that would match HIV commodity usage data against procurement performance, which would help to indicate their effects on continuity and effectiveness within the context of HIV testing and counselling services.

Service Delivery

Service delivery encompasses a range of activities including the assessment, strategic planning, and monitoring and evaluation of a programme. Models of service delivery will vary according to local, regional, and national requirements. Assessment of service delivery will include determining the current and required infrastructure, situation analysis, site readiness, staff selection, referral networks, and phasing and time frame for implementation and scaling up of HIV testing and counselling services. Strategic planning will include developing site selection criteria, client registration and intake, testing protocols, counselling protocols, informed consent, disclosure, lab protocols, integration with other HIV/AIDS initiatives, establishing referral networks, and post test care. Monitoring and evaluation will include service accessibility, site monitoring, evaluation of testing techniques, adequacy of protocols, patient flow, referral use, and various methods of quality assurance.

HIV testing and counselling must be scaled up in order to meet the increasing demand for access to treatment, care and prevention services. While the guiding principles of traditional VCT models remain, scaling up will require a change of approach to a more routine and widespread public health approach. HIV testing and counselling should be offered as standard practice:

i) when requested to assist in the prevention of transmission or acquisition of HIV,
ii) where medically indicated in the context of clinical care, and
iii) for the prevention of transmission from mothers to children.

The minimum acceptable standards for HIV testing and counselling approaches requires all models of service delivery respect the following principles:

i) HIV testing and counselling should be voluntary.
ii) Individuals should have sufficient information, understanding and freedom of choice to give informed consent for testing.
iii) Pre-test information should describe the purpose and procedure of HIV testing, and the treatment and support that will be available after testing.
iv) There should be appropriate post-test information, counselling and/or referral.
v) Those who test positive should receive counselling and referral to care, support and treatment, where available.
vi) HIV test results and counselling records should be treated confidentially and only those health care workers with a

direct role in the management of patients should have access to this information.

vii) Those who test negative should receive counselling support to enable them to remain free of HIV.

Models of Service Delivery

The present provision of HIV testing and counselling is frequently based in stand-alone community and hospital-based centres offering standard, individualised voluntary counselling and testing and employing ELISA technology.

Present HIV testing and counselling approaches include the following:

Model 1. Individual pre- and post-test counselling and testing ("classic" model, most free-standing VCT sites).

Model 2. Group information, opt-in individual pre-test counselling, individual post-test counselling

Model 3. Group information, opt-out individual testing, individual post-test counselling for seropositives, seronegatives are informed of their negative status.

Model 4. Group information, opt-in couple/family pre-test counselling, individual/couple/family post-test counselling (shared confidentiality model).

Model 5. No pre-test information, screening/testing (with an option to opt-out), individual post-test counselling for those found HIV+ (screening of STI attendees, drug treatment programme attendees and women attending antenatal clinics)

Model 6. Mandatory testing

Model 7. Counselling without testing

HIV testing and counselling services are best supported through approaches that are based on integrated HIV/AIDS care, treatment, support and prevention. The rate of HIV testing and counselling uptake may become inextricably linked with access to ARV treatment, as individuals may be encouraged to find out their HIV status if they have access to better treatment options. Rapid scaling up of care also requires a diversification and expansion of HIV testing and counselling services linked to clinical care and ANC settings. This requires various approaches towards HIV testing and counselling implementation including:

i) Use of HIV rapid tests in treatment settings situated away from provincial treatment centres and in areas of high prevalence and vulnerability to HIV
ii) Diversification of sites where testing and counselling can be provided, e.g., rapid testing to be situated in those areas where vulnerable populations may be greatest, for example, STI/reproductive health care services, TB services, IDU services, and in non-clinical areas where prevention may be optimised, such as antenatal care and young people services
iii) Outreach and mobile initiatives may be necessary to improve access to HIV testing and counselling among 'hard to reach' groups, e.g., IDUs, sex workers, young people
iv) Although there may be different approaches to service delivery within countries and between countries, the principles of the recommended public health approach for scaling up HIV testing and counselling should be common to the varying approaches.

As the number of people seeking HIV care, treatment and prevention is rapidly increasing, there is an urgent need to provide decentralised services to cope with this demand and improve access. Services should therefore be implemented in ways that address this need for decentralisation and embraces a range of approaches for delivering testing and counselling including community or district-based delivery approaches.

Planning Service Delivery

Planning for the following will help to determine the service delivery approach in terms of where HIV testing and counselling will be provided, how it will be provided and who will be involved:

i) Clarify infrastructure needs: current and required; Is it a new service or an addition to existing service?

ii) What different preparatory activities, staff roles and responsibilities are required?

Situation analysis including epidemiology, geographic mapping of testing and counselling facilities, referral sites and networks HIV testing and counselling uptake:

i) *Assess health-seeking behaviour*: Whether individuals understand the need for care, treatment and prevention and where they choose or are able to access this.

ii) *Assess various models of service delivery*: Flexibility in models of service delivery will be required to ensure responsiveness of the planned service to target groups, health systems in place and context.

iii) *Determine linkages and referral mechanisms to provide additional services*: Determine capacity of referral sites to take on additional clients.

iv) Determine training and resource needs of testing and counselling service and referral sites.

v) Determine management structure for staff and human resource, financial, service delivery approach, and commodities.

Ensuring access requires community mobilisation to increase uptake of services and address barriers such as lack of information or understanding, stigma and marginalisation, and affordability Phasing and time frame for implementation and scaling up; plans for resources to be in place.

Operational Issues

Components of service delivery that must be addressed in order to provide quality testing and counselling programmes include:

i) Clarifying requirements for staff, space, equipment and supplies
ii) Staffing and human resource management
iii) Standardised protocols and patient selection
iv) Linkages to other services for post-test support and involving a range of stakeholders especially people with HIV
v) Raising awareness of the benefits and availability of testing and counselling
vi) Strategies to address stigma and discrimination
vii) Monitoring and evaluation (M&E)

Clarifying requirements for staff, space, equipment and supplies: Estimating requirements for space, equipment, supplies, and staff. The requirements for setting up stand-alone or integrated testing and counselling services will vary. Factors to consider will include the setting, volume of clients expected, staffing availability, testing protocols adopted, and equipment, supplies and infrastructure available. Infrastructure will be needed, including private counselling space and waiting areas, counselling rooms, and a testing area. Other supplies will include HIV test kits, condoms, gloves and other medical supplies, including those for universal precautions, PEP blister packs for accidental exposure, sharps disposal containers, contaminated waste containers, and disinfectant.

The staffing requirements will vary depending on the volume expected but all individuals providing HIV testing and counselling services whether on a paid or volunteer basis must have adequate training to perform these duties in a professional and credible manner that will ensure quality of service and allow for clients to feel confidence in the skills and discretion of staff.

Staffing and human resource management: Human resources are the most critical component of HIV testing and counselling services. A commitment is required at all levels to develop and support human resources. Many different types of human resources are needed for the effective delivery of HIV testing and counselling services including people with skills in management, administration, supply management, clinical care and community-based care. Health care staff groups and volunteers can be trained in the core principles and delivery of testing and counselling services.

Training in HIV, testing and counselling services core competencies and skills should be included as a module in the training curricula of all physicians, nurses, social workers and other health care staff. All counsellors and other staff should participate in ongoing training and supervision. Provision of clear job descriptions, lines of management, codes of conduct, case conferences, staff meetings, and programme vision and goals will be required.

Training, supervision, and support will help to decrease attrition and staff burn-out, maintain staff motivation, and facilitate dealing with equity and stigma within the workplace. The content, appropriateness and delivery of training for different staff groups will depend on the allocated role and responsibilities based on the service delivery approach. The content of training should be based on standard treatment protocols and clinical management guidelines.

Standardisation of training and developing guidelines for accreditation of counsellors is a way of ensuring quality of service and follow-up of training. Building skills and competencies through training should be linked to opportunities to use the skills in practice. Evaluation of training and continuing education need to be budgeted for and supported. Networking and developing links for staff with other providers and with national counselling networks where they exist should also be developed to ensure quality standards in testing and counselling.

Health care workers are also among those affected by HIV/AIDS. The impact of HIV on staff can increase staff turnover and adversely affect staff morale and their ability to perform in their jobs. Providing a safe working environment includes workplace programmes for HIV prevention, treatment, psychosocial support, management of violence and assault, and also availability of PEP, Hepatitis B vaccination, and UP for staff. These are important measures for addressing the impact of HIV/AIDS on health care workers. Health care workers should benefit from the available HIV treatment services so that their ability to perform their job is not adversely affected.

Standardised protocols and quality standards: Clear operational policies, quality standards, and protocols are required for service delivery including protocols for:

i) client selection
ii) client registration and intake
iii) delivery of HIV testing and counselling
iv) PEP
v) laboratory protocols
vi) pre-test counselling
vii) obtaining informed consent
viii) maintaining confidentiality
ix) beneficial disclosure
x) post-test counselling, care and support
xi) ensuring non-discrimination of service provision
xii) referral mechanisms

Protocols and monitoring procedures should be regularly reviewed and used for training of health care workers. Information management systems will be needed for monitoring of client registration, intake and referral that maintain confidentiality and can be used to reconfigure services and protocols as required. Quality improvement processes are required for auditing adherence to policies, protocols and procedures. It is important to use these processes to assess issues such as staff competency, counsellor skills, counselling protocols, laboratory testing adequacy, and the client perspective on the accessibility and acceptability of testing and counselling services.

Linkages to other services: Comprehensive HIV testing and counselling services should be delivered as part of a package of prevention, treatment, care and support interventions. This will involve close linkages to community members and structures including post-test clubs, NGOs, CBOs, private and public health providers, traditional healers, and people with HIV. Effective referral networks are necessary between the range of stakeholders and services at health facility and community level to achieve continuity of care, treatment and prevention and to meet the range of needs of people accessing testing and counselling and the needs of people with HIV.

Linking and integrating with other health services can include, for example, those for prevention of HIV in infants and young children, ARV treatment, STI, TB, family planning, and paediatric care. Care must be taken to refer people to good quality services.

Raising awareness of the benefits and availability of HIV Testing and Counselling Increasing access to HIV testing and counselling involves raising awareness of the accessibility of services and the benefits of individuals knowing their HIV status. This includes increasing awareness of the benefits from advances in the prevention of HIV infection including MTCT and treatment of HIV-related diseases including ARV treatment where available.

Reducing barriers to access to HIV testing and counselling services for vulnerable populations such as women, young people, sex workers, MSM, IDUs, refugees, and prison populations will be an important consideration for service delivery. Strategies to raise awareness and promote uptake of services can include outreach and peer based methods to mobilise community. Cost sharing and financial arrangements to encourage vulnerable groups to use services may also increase uptake. HIV testing and counselling services must be developed in ways that respond to the specific needs of these populations.

Evidence shows that stigma and discrimination prevent people from accessing HIV testing, counselling, care, treatment and prevention. Involvement of a range of stakeholders including healthcare workers, communities, post-test clubs and people with HIV can contribute significantly to reducing stigma and to providing a supportive environment for people accessing HIV testing and counselling services and for people with HIV. NGOs, CBOs, post-test clubs and people with HIV also play an important role in providing information and education and in working with service providers to increase the coverage and use of services. Community education efforts also help create a more supportive environment for treatment, care and prevention programmes.

Monitoring and evaluation: The goal of monitoring and evaluation of HIV testing and counselling services is:

i) to increase the efficiency, effectiveness and quality of services delivered by providers
ii) to improve the availability, accessibility, acceptability and use of testing and counselling services by users

An important objective of monitoring and evaluation is to provide managers and decisionmakers with the information to improve or scale up service delivery. HIV testing and counselling services should consider developing monitoring and evaluation as part of the planning process. Monitoring and evaluation will strengthen the quality of the service. It will include methods to assess service accessibility, site monitoring, country evaluation of testing techniques, adequacy of protocols, activity levels and patient flow including all interactions from entry to exit of counselling and testing services, ethical guidelines, referral use, return rates, and follow-up, and various methods of quality assurance.

Critical issues for scaling up HIV testing and counselling service delivery:

i) *Integration of HIV testing and counselling services with other health care services.* Testing and counselling services can be successfully integrated with other health care, support, and prevention services including home based and community care programmes. These services can include ARV and HIV treatment and care, and FP, STI, TB and PMTCT/ANC services.

ii) *Ensuring services actually reach those most in need.* Testing and counselling services should be developed to enable access to vulnerable populations including, for example, women, young people, sex workers, migrants, rural populations, mobile populations, MSM, and prison populations. The development of testing and counselling resources and protocols to meet the needs of different populations will be required.

iii) *Issues for scaling up testing and counselling services.* Rapid scaling up of testing and counselling requires ensuring that quality standards continue to be met within services. Flexible service models are required that will be specific to the context and region. A major challenge will be to ensure that human resource development is sufficient for scaling up testing and counselling service delivery including paid staff, volunteers, peer and outreach staff.

Capacity Building and Training

The scaling up of HIV testing and counselling services requires effective capacity building and training to ensure that services are of consistently high quality and that they meet the needs of the communities they serve. Capacity building is a concept that goes beyond training and attainment of skills. It includes the strengthening of organisations and systems, and establishing and supporting linkages and networks. Training and support for all cadres of staff are essential components of capacity building. The capacity building and training requirements of counselling and testing services will vary depending on the setting and services offered. Central co-ordination is recommended to build and support capacity for the effective running and development of a counselling and testing service or programme. This could be achieved by appointing a full-time National counselling and testing co-ordinator, and using the expertise of a counselling and testing steering committee. The steering committee could be comprise people with skills in:

i) Monitoring and evaluation for progress and quality assurance
ii) Training
iii) Finance
iv) Policy
v) Logistics
vi) Laboratory expertise
vii) Counselling
viii) Data management

These people may already be in place and working with ARV, MTCT, and TB programmes. This would facilitate linkages and collaborations with these programmes. Different countries have developed different approaches and models for providing counselling and testing services. If NGOs have a significant role in delivering services, it would be important to include them at this central level.

The counselling and testing coordinator and committee would:

i) Assess the capacity building and training requirements at local, district and national levels that are necessary to carry out development and scaling up of counselling and testing services

ii) Develop a capacity building and training strategy

iii) Review existing training materials

iv) Review available capacity building and training expertise

v) Utilise existing institutions to provide skills and support to management and staff, such as counsellors and laboratory personnel

vi) Monitor progress and quality of service development.

The committee would include:

i) Technical experts in HIV testing and counselling

ii) Communications experts for publicity and advocacy

iii) Data managers involved in service delivery and monitoring and evaluation

iv) Logistics and supplies experts

v) Community development expertise.

Capacity Building

Capacity must be developed at all levels to ensure that all counselling and testing services:

i) *Develop in a coordinated way:* In many countries there are a wide number of public, NGO and private counselling and testing providers. Encouraging these different providers to share experiences, resources and challenges can be beneficial, enabling them to learn from each other.

ii) *Reach different population groups and different geographical areas:* In many countries services are confined to large urban areas. As a result, vulnerable population groups with special needs may not have access to services. Such groups include young people, prisoners, sex workers, migrant workers, internally displaced persons (IDP) and IDUs.

iii) *Support quality control of HIV testing and counselling:* National guidelines on testing policy and practice and a national quality assurance system will help to guarantee that testing is carried out in a consistent way and to the highest standard. Development of standards practice for counselling training and selection may help to raise the quality of counselling.

iv) *Enable bulk purchase of commodities:* Central co-ordination of purchasing and distributing commodities such as testing kits, condoms and HIV education material may cut down on costs and increase the reliability of supply chains. Institutional capacity building to develop and provide HIV testing and counselling services is important in order to allow the capacity of current institutions to scale up; the capacity of an area to support a new service and training of managerial staff at this level.

Training Requirements

Basic training is essential for all HIV testing and counselling staff members, including reception and administrative staff. Some areas will be common to all staff members, but particular sub groups will need additional technical training. Training needs for counselling and testing staff include:

i) *Basic counselling training (pre-service and in-service)*: All counsellors will need basic training for routine cases. This training would include:

   a) Pre-test education/pre-test counselling

   b) Post-test counselling

   c) Ongoing counselling

ii) *Advanced/specialised counselling training:* Some counsellors in the services can be trained in more advanced counselling skills, so that they can support less experienced counsellors with complex cases, or have clients/patients referred to them. Specialised counselling training will also be needed for counsellors seeing young people, families/couples and vulnerable groups such as sex workers and IDUs. This training may include counselling for areas such as domestic violence and rape and pre-marital/couple counselling.

iii) *Training of trainers*: In many settings a rapid scaling up of HIV testing and counselling services is planned and training of trainers is essential for this.

iv) *Continuing education*: HIV testing and counselling is a rapidly changing field. For example, new ARV treatment and PMTCT opportunities mean that there are huge benefits to knowing one's status. Counsellors will need continuing education so that they are aware of current treatment options and, for example, areas such as infant feeding counselling if they are involved in PMTCT. Staff who are involved in HIV testing will also need to have access to continuing education so that they can be aware of new test kits, technologies and procedures.

v) *Ongoing supervision, support and mentoring*. Burn-out and staff attrition have been noted in many HIV testing and counselling services. A senior counsellor will need training to enable him/her to develop a programme of support, supervision and mentoring for counsellors. Regular staff appraisals can help to keep staff motivated and maintain a high quality of service.

vi) *Monitoring and evaluation:* Monitoring and evaluation is important to assess the effectiveness of the training and counselling services, and for future planning.

Training of counsellors: If significantly greater access to counselling and testing services is to be achieved, counsellors from a wider range of backgrounds must be trained. Choice of counsellor type will depend on different country circumstances and needs. The content of basic counselling training may be similar for all cadres of counsellors, but may be tailored to the educational background and previous experience of the counsellor/counsellor group. Counsellors may include people from the following groups:

i) *Traditional counsellors*: with a health/social work background School leavers/counsellors with secondary school education have been recruited in some settings, particularly in countries where there is a lack of tertiary education facilities and high unemployment for school leavers. People with HIV — in many settings people with HIV—have been trained as counsellors. They can offer particularly valuable services and help to support others who test HIV positive. However, people with HIV working as counsellors may themselves be vulnerable to work-related stress and burnout and will need careful support and supervision to avoid this Retired professionals. Retired health workers, teachers and preachers often already have counselling skills and hold the trust of their community. They can often work part-time or cover out-of-hours services.

ii) *Community/peer counsellors*: Community counsellors, who are often without formal education but are respected members of the community with wide life experience—mothers, for example—can sometimes offer ongoing support to people following HIV testing and counselling.

Training of HIV testing staff: Away from clinic/hospital settings, non-laboratory staff will often carry out testing. Training will be needed for:

i) *Facility-based staff*, to take samples and perform rapid tests.

ii) *Laboratory staff*, to perform confirmatory tests and assist with training of facility-based testing staff. Linkages to reference laboratory services for routine quality control will also need to be set up.

The following issues should be considered in planning for staff capacity building and training needs:

i) *Staff recruitment (*lab, counsellors, testing staff, etc.)

  a) Decision of whom to recruit (motivation, roles and responsibilities, background)

  b) Formulating job descriptions (duties and responsibilities)

  c) Identification of staff support requirements.

ii) *Staff retention*: Retaining already trained counselling and testing staff can be a major challenge. High staff turnover is costly, inefficient and may result in low morale for remaining staff. The following areas should be reviewed to prevent staff attrition and burn-out:

  a) *Salaries* (consider local factors, such as the salary scales of similar programmes)

  b) *HIV/AIDS morbidity and mortality* including emotional needs and addressing stigma. This can be addressed through: support for HIV workplace policy development; HIV education and support programmes for staff and families; access to HIV testing and counselling for all staff and families; access to health care and universal prevention/infection control.

iii) *Mobility issues*: Many HIV testing and counselling services report high turnover of staff, with qualified/trained staff moving to other posts. Other HIV testing and counselling services have reported difficulties recruiting staff to rural or remote areas. The following ways of retaining staff could be considered:

  a) Incentives

  b) Career structure

  c) Professional development

  d) Continuing medical education

  e) Differential between urban and rural work

  f) Implementation of policies and creation of environments to discourage active recruitment of well qualified staff to other countries and, in parallel, encourage placement of new graduates.

iv) *Stress and psychological management*

a) Provision of ongoing supervision, support and mentoring

b) Provision of a supportive working environment, e.g., coffee breaks

c) Role recognition

d) Reduction/modification of workload

e) Facilitation of flexible and part-time working

f) Development of a staff appraisal system, including recognition of different roles and feedback to staff Sympathetic consideration of performance issues due to burn out.

g) Provision of a programme of staff development and in-service training.

Critical issues of capacity building and training for scaling up HIV testing and counselling include:

i) *Counselling for other vulnerable populations:* There is a lack of training materials for IDU, sex workers, migrants and IDPs, prisoners and incarcerated populations and young people.

ii) *Advanced counselling:* This includes counselling for, for example, discordant couples, suicidal clients, rape victims, domestic violence and child sex abuse

iii) *Training institution resources:* Some high prevalence countries have other development challenges, such as lack of education infrastructure and corresponding lack of expertise within the country to carry out capacity building and training. This is particularly acute for countries coming out of conflict.

iv) *Selecting appropriate staff for training*: This can be a particular problem when selecting staff members for in-depth training or training opportunities abroad.

v) *Mainstreaming HIV counselling training*: This includes counselling and HIV testing training in other curricula, e.g. medical school, religious institutional training, teacher training college, nursing, etc.

Management and Coordination

Scaling up HIV testing and counselling services requires an effective system of management and coordination to ensure that policies, guidelines, systems, resources, roles and responsibilities and deadlines are translated into programme activities and implemented to achieve HIV testing and counselling service delivery as equitably as possible.

Management and coordination will vary depending on the setting. Coordination is important for ensuring quality of HIV testing and counselling services and links to other services, efficiency of HIV testing and counselling services, and better use of resources to reduce duplication of services. Communication between managers is essential to achieve these aims.

At the national level, the management system should be defined during the planning of HIV testing and counselling services, ensuring that it has the capacity and resources for co-ordination and making connections between policies, decision making and implementation. Management functions can be carried out at different levels and may be centralised or decentralised depending on the degree of delegation possible within different operational settings. Leadership requires a clear vision for the programme and for quality of care.

The major functions of the management system for HIV testing and counselling services include:

i) An advisory function, responsible for addressing policy issues regarding the implementation of HIV testing and counselling services
ii) Day-to-day management for implementation of HIV testing and counselling services

iii) Monitoring and evaluation

iv) Co-ordination within HIV testing and counselling services, with other relevant services and with other 'external' stakeholders.

A formal advisory body whose tasks are to support the management system and advise on policy issues should carry out the advisory function. Membership of the advisory body should include health professionals directly involved in the programme, 'user' representatives, professional bodies, social security and other providers of services such as insurance companies and employers. Where possible HIV testing and counselling services should be integrated within ARV treatment and care programmes.

Issues that an advisory body would address include:

i) national policy formulation on provision of HIV testing and counselling, including financing and phased approach

ii) development of country-specific practical guidelines

iii) estimation or assessment of scale of HIV testing and counselling services required

iv) selection of clinics/sites suitable for the provision of HIV testing and counselling services

v) capacity building for clinicians, counsellors, testing technicians at identified sites

vi) development of process indicators and evaluation tools

vii) dissemination of information on the impact of HIV testing and counselling services.

The day-to-day project management function of testing and counselling services requires overseeing different service-related and administrative aspects of the programme, such as capacity building, procurement and distribution, monitoring and evaluation, and finance.

Management can be provided within an existing health system or established prior to the implementation of new testing and counselling services. Management systems can also be implemented within overall HIV strategy. An effective management system will clearly define lines of authority, communication, and roles and responsibilities at different levels. Managers will require ongoing training programmes using existing training institutions. Responsibilities of managers may include:

a) Ensuring that service providers are familiar with minimum standards for HIV testing and counselling services and procedures of service delivery on an ongoing basis
b) Linking government services with other providers and services
c) Facilitating positive institutional and service provider attitudes aimed at reducing stigma and discrimination amongst health care providers. This could be done through on-going training.
d) Provision of management systems for information and data management for decision making
e) Implementing a monitoring and evaluation strategy for testing and counselling services and implementation with clear defined indicators and implementation plan
f) Monitoring of goals, targets and achievements to demonstrate success and facilitate trust which included reporting systems for local and global requirements
g) Familiarity with costing of HIV testing and counselling services and resource management
h) Establishing referral networks
i) Assuring quality, accountability, and transparency
j) Provision of ongoing communication, job plans and feedback, training, supervision, and system of support, investment and motivation to programme staff to minimise attrition.

The scaling up process within HIV/AIDS programmes an services requires a shift from a centralised approach to a decentralised mechanisms of planning and implementation that include a broader range of factors for the different components of an HIV/AIDS programme. HIV testing and counselling services can be implemented in a number of sectors and certain aspects of scaling up through a more decentralised approach can apply here. Strong central coordination and capacity at local levels is required, but the focus of the central management function in a decentralised approach is more on the setting of policies and programme parameters, financing of projects, facilitation and training, and monitoring and evaluation, rather than implementation, which takes place at decentralised levels.

Coordination

Coordination of testing and counselling services comprises the following:

i) Coordination of different programmes for delivering HIV testing and counselling services. The use of standardised protocols for provision of HIV testing and counselling services will ensure that common standards are met, support the efficiency of programmes, and avoid duplication. This is especially important if programmes are to build on existing experience, pilot projects, and other small-scale experiences.

ii) Coordination of HIV testing and counselling services with other AIDS activities and other health sector undertakings such as the Global Fund Country Coordinating mechanism, and the national strategic plan. This would also help to ensure integration within health care systems.

iv) Coordination of activities between the central and implementation levels is also critical for effective management, to share expertise, and to ensure effective service delivery. This is because different but inextricably linked activities will take place at different levels, e.g., procurement of essential commodities at the central level while provision of HIV testing and counselling services is at the implementation level.

Critical issues for management and coordination of HIV testing and counselling services are:

i) *Management resources:* Identifying and defining leadership within testing and counselling services is a key task for programme developers. This will include establishing clear guidelines on management and operational systems for scaling up HIV testing and counselling services. Adequate resources are required for provision of current and projected management systems for scaling up testing and counselling services.
ii) *Management training*: Identifying opportunities for enhancing managerial skills and training will be required for scaling up HIV testing and counselling services. Key tasks include identifying who to train and to what level of management. The development of support systems and supervision for managers is also required.
iii) *Quality assurance*: In order to minimise wastage and duplication, improved coordination is required between partner agencies, managers, service providers and beneficiaries of services; this will result in better use of resources, sharing of expertise, improve quality, efficiency, and all components that would enhance scaling up of testing and counselling services. Development of appropriate indicators to monitor HIV testing and counselling services is required, including the use of effective information management systems.
iv) *Human resources management*: Human resource management is a major challenge for scaling up testing and counselling services. For example, how to avoid high staff attrition rates in staff and counsellors, how to increase number of trained staff and volunteers to meet

requirements for scaling up. Issues to consider will include ensuring that adequate resources, training, and support are available for staff including access to HIV testing and counselling services and health care.

Costs and Financing

When planning HIV testing and counselling services it is essential to have accurate cost estimates. To implement and scale up it is necessary to secure adequate financing for all aspects of the programme. Failure to predict realistic costs and secure sufficient funding has sometimes led to existing counselling and testing services not being able to scale up to meet demand. The costing and financing requirements of counselling and testing services will vary depending on the setting and services offered.

Estimating costs for a counselling and testing programme requires detailed data about the number of people who are expected to access services, the planned components of the service and the costs of these components. Estimating programme costs entails:

i) defining programme targets (number of people expected to access testing and/or related services)
ii) estimating start up and ongoing costs for the site/s
iii) estimating start up and ongoing cost for all cadres of staff
iv) estimating any potential income generated by the programme (cost sharing/cost recovery, etc.).

There will be differing cost and financing needs depending on the site chosen. For example integrating counselling and testing into existing health services (ANC, TB, STI) or adding counselling and testing to community organisations or stand-alone sites. When planning a counselling and testing programme and/or writing funding proposals it is important not to underestimate costs, particularly initial start-up costs. It is also a good idea to include a contingency in the budget to cover unexpected expenditure.

The following are key challenges in preparing budgets:

i) *Lack of data when making projections and predictions*: This can be a particular challenge when setting up a service as it can be difficult to anticipate how many people will attend HIV testing and counselling services, how may people from different populations groups will attend and numbers of people requiring follow-up services.

ii) Means and ways of justifying costs and budgets

iii) *Inflation and exchange rates*: Many developing countries have high inflation or fluctuating exchange rates. This may make it difficult to budget for both expenditure within the country and for consumables which are purchased outside the country. It is therefore important to make realistic predictions for inflation with a stated margin of error. Donor agencies may also have regulations about currencies in which budgets should be made and state exchange rates.

iv) *Unplanned activities*: Even when the most careful plans and budgets have been made there will often be additional activities which require funding and other unplanned expenses. This is a particular problem for new HIV testing and counselling services. However even for well-established services circumstances may change. For example, one HIV testing and counselling site had relied on supplies of free condoms from another NGO. When this NGO no longer provided condoms they had to purchase these from the central medical stores. A contingency for these unplanned expenses should be made in the budget. Some donor agencies may be reluctant to agree to contingency budget lines but will respond by providing additional funding if circumstances change.

vi) *Competition with other programmes and organisations for donor resources*: Despite an increased emphasis on funding for HIV activities with new funding mechanisms like the global fund there is still huge competition for limited funds. Participation in coordinating funding approaches such as the CCMs may facilitate accessing funds. Furthermore this can help organisations providing or planning to provide counselling and testing to form linkages with other HIV support organisations that can provide ongoing care and support following HIV testing and counselling services, community based advocacy work and legal services. For example linkages with groups of people with HIV, health services providers, condom social marketing programmes, church and faith based groups and other community groups will enhance counselling and testing services and may reduce costs as support services may be available, provided by these organisations.

Financing

Funding requirements will differ widely depending on the country and context. There is a wide range of options for funding. Many counselling and testing sites will receive funding from a combination of sources. The major funding sources are:

i) *Local and central government*: Many integrated and national programmes may be fully funded by government funding and be part of an integrated comprehensive HIV programme. In other settings the government may provide some funding or may supply and fund or second staff or pay or supply commodities such as test kits.

ii) *Bilateral and multilateral donors*: Bilateral and multilateral donors remain a major source of funding for HIV interventions in most developing countries. Accessing funds depends on local criteria.

iii) *International agencies and foundations*: The global fund has become a major source of new funding for HIV interventions. Government or NGOs can access funding for counselling and testing through the country coordinating mechanism.

iv) *Private sector*: Increasingly workplaces are considering offering counselling and testing as part of workplace medical schemes or will fund counselling and testing for their workforce at independent counselling and testing sites. Private medical services often offer HIV testing with or without counselling to clients. In this circumstance the client will pay the full cost of HIV testing, making it beyond the reach of some people.

v) *User fees/cost recovery*: Some NGOs have a system of charging clients a small fee for HIV testing and counselling services. This usually is a fraction of the actual costs and in practice does not contribute significantly to the costs of the service.

vi) *Local fundraising*: Some counselling and testing services may have the opportunity to attract funds by local fund-raising or raise funds by providing training or other services for other organisations or renting out facilities and services to other organisations when not in use.

Because of the complexities of funding sources and mechanisms in many countries it can often be cost-effective to employ someone whose responsibility is to source and secure funding. Some counselling and testing programmes employ resource mobilisers who are knowledgeable about funding sources and are experts in preparing funding applications. Resource mobiliser tasks may include:

— Identify funding sources, both local and international.
— Ascertain, for each funding source, areas of focus and interest of the donor, funding cycles and deadlines.
— Prepare proposals with clear strategic plan and budget tailored to the donor's interests.
— Explore ways of being represented on the country co-ordinating mechanism (CCM) to facilitate access to funding.

— Co-ordinate, with other team members, donor reporting to ensure that reports are on time and in line with donor requirements to ensure continuing and future funding.

— Document past successes and disseminate widely. Funders often want to support programmes that have already demonstrated that they are effective, acceptable and successful.

— Arrange dissemination workshops and presentations at meetings and conferences.

Skills needed in costing and financing for HIV testing and counselling services include:

— *Management*: Management training will be needed to support the accounting and finance staff and to co-ordinate financial systems and processes.

— *Proposal writing*: A key part of any project proposal is to ensure that the budget is as accurate and realistic as possible and that it is presented in a consistent way.

— *Accounting*: Accounting training will be needed, but this will vary depend on the site. The method and complexity of accounting will depend on the size and scope of HIV testing and counselling services and the reporting required by donors and government.

— *Inventory control*: Basic inventory control skills are needed in all training and counselling sites to ensure consistent supply of consumables such as test kits, condoms, etc., and to provide a check against possible loss or theft.

REFERENCES

"Candle of hope: the AIDS programme of the Thai Red Cross", *Strategies for Hope Series,* No. 9. London: ActionAid, 1994.

"Commodity Management in VCT Programmes: A Planning Guide", FHI/MSH-RPM, 2003.

Counselling for HIV/AIDS: a key to caring. For policy-makers, planners and implementors of counselling activities, Geneva: WHO, 1995.

Dhaliwal, Mandeep, etal, *Scaling up HIV Testing and Counselling Services a toolkit for programme managers*, International HIV/ AIDS Alliance, 2003.

From Principle to Practice: Greater Involvement of People Living with or Affected by HIV/AIDS (GIPA)", September 1999.

Government of India, *National AIDS Contol Programme, HIV Testing Policy,* 1995.

Increasing Access to HIV Testing and Counselling, WHO, 2002.

Interim TB-HIV Guidelines, WHO, 2003.

Joint United Nations Programme on HIV/AIDS, *Counselling and HIV/AIDS: UNAIDS Technical Update,* November, 1997 .

"Keys to Counselling", *AIDS Action Newsletter*, Issue 24. London: AHRTAG, 1994.

Opening the HIV/AIDS epidemic – Guidance of encouraging beneficial disclosure, ethical partner counselling &appropriate use of HIV case reporting, UNAIDS, 2001.

Opening the HIV/AIDS epidemic – Guidance of encouraging beneficial disclosure, ethical partner counselling &appropriate use of HIV case reporting, UNAIDS, 2001.

Sittitrai W., *Reproductive health and HIV/AIDS. Myanmar training manual: a community-based approach for youth and women*, Yangon, UNICEF, 1995.

Source book for HIV/AIDS counselling training, Geneva: WHO, 1994.

The Right to Know: New Approaches in HIV Testing and Counselling. WHO, 2003.

UNAIDS policy on HIV testing and counselling, Geneva: UNAIDS, 1997.

Voluntary Counselling and Testing (VCT), Paper for the UNAIDS expert panel on HIV testing in UN peacekeeping operations, 2001.

Voluntary Counselling and Testing (VCT): Program tools for implementing VCT, CDC, *Global AIDS Program,* April, 2003.

"World Bank Technical Guide for Procurement of HIV/AIDS Medicines and Related Supplies", *Draft*, 2003.

4

Ethical Partner Counselling

Effective counselling is important in helping people with concerns about sexuality, STI and HIV. Many people feel unable to talk about them because of embarrassment or fear of rejection. If they do, they may not receive the emotional support, information and skills they require. Fears about the future, guilt, anger and despair may overwhelm them. They may not feel able to talk to their partner about sexual problems, safer sex or an STI/HIV diagnosis. These situations are complex and clients need time to talk them over and make good decisions.

Counselling is different from providing a medical service where providers generally give treatment, health information, advice and instructions to service users. This partnership model means that attitudes are very important in counselling. The counsellor's attitudes as a counsellor are very important. Sexuality is a sensitive subject and unless the counsellor show the clients that she/he care about and respect them, they will not be able to talk openly about their lives and feelings.

Counselling empowers individuals to prevent transmission of HIV by enabling them to cope with the personal implications of an HIV diagnosis and to make informed personal decisions, including those related to sexuality and reproduction. Counsellors should provide psychosocial and spiritual support to those who are affected and should assist clients to make decisions that will improve the quality of their lives. Counsellors can help the affected persons adopt new lifestyles, and assist them to retain their identities, independence, privacy, social status and self-worth. This can then reduce the risk of negative outcomes, re-infection, and transmission of infection to others.

MODELS OF COUNSELLING

There are several models of counselling where the counsellor can use his skills. GATHER is one that is often used in contraceptive counselling.

Greet the clients

Ask the clients why they have come and about their situations

Tell the clients how you can help them

Help the clients to make their own decisions

Explain how to use the methods they have chosen

Return visits are arranged to see how they are getting on.

This model was designed for contraceptive counselling, but counsellor can adapt it for STI/HIV.

REDA is another model, which is more open and flexible.

Rapport is developed between counsellor and client

Explore the problem, situation and options for change

Decide on the best option

Act on the decision.

ROLE OF COUNSELLORS

Counsellors have many opportunities to counsel clients on other sexual and reproductive health issues, including STI/HIV because:

— Counsellors see people who are in sexual relationships and may be at risk of STI/HIV.

— Counsellors distribute male and female condoms, the only methods that protect against STI/HIV.

— Clients need protection from unwanted pregnancy and STI/HIV.

— Clients need to take risk of STI/HIV into account when they make a decision about which contraceptive to use.

— Some counsellors are used to talking about sexual issues.

— Counsellors may talk about gender relations, which affect risk of STI/HIV.

— Counsellors can discuss concerns about STI, including signs and symptoms and refer.

— Counsellors can be aware of the possibility of sexual abuse and support clients.

Some providers worry that integrating STI/HIV into their family planning programme will have a negative impact on their services. In fact it may improve quality for the following reasons:

— The client is looked at in a holistic way, which helps the client with family planning and sexual life generally. Clients feel that the counsellor cares about them as people rather than contraceptive acceptors.

— The use of existing facilities is maximised because counsellors are already trained, experienced and trusted.

— The counsellor can reach a wider group of clients with unmet needs, including young people, men and those not at risk of pregnancy.

— Having a package of different health services helps to prevent stigma.

— The services may have more access to government and other support services, including traditional healers.

There are some differences between counselling on family planning and counselling on STI/HIV, which the counsellor need to address in his plan to integrate services. It is important to use a participatory process in which leaders, managers and staff at all levels explore the costs and benefits of integrating different types of sexual health services into the existing programmes. The counsellor then has to make a joint decision on which services, if any, to offer in relation to local needs and service gaps and values, identity and resources.

The counsellor may feel that STI/HIV counselling is an additional task that reveals problems that are difficult to resolve. He/she need to take part in the decision to integrate STI/HIV counselling, given a chance to express his/her fears and to identify the support needs. People may see family planning clinics as places where 'respectable' married women go for contraception, to do with fertility, not talking about a potentially fatal disease passed through sex. The counsellor may fear that the change of image will drive away clients.

Counsellors need knowledge of the medical and a social issues of HIV and contacts with the family and community to address them. There is more stigma, judgmental attitudes and secrecy around STI/HIV than family planning. This makes it harder to talk about openly and the consequences of disclosure more difficult. Counsellors have limited ways to help clients with these issues. It is important to work for changes in attitudes towards STI/HIV, perhaps by collaborating with other organisations.

The counsellor need knowledge of available resources for STI/HIV prevention, support and care in the locality. Offer all existing clients the opportunity for STI/HIV prevention counselling. The counsellor might make the services more accessible to groups who are also vulnerable to STI/HIV, such as young people, men or single women. He/she may need to change his/her image and to attract these groups and provide them with confidential, acceptable services. If couples agree, it can be helpful to counsel them together. This can build trust, help them to communicate more easily and make joint decisions about HIV testing and safer sex options.

People who are motivated to counsel are more likely to make good, empathetic counsellors. Managers should only give counselling duties to providers who feel committed to it. The counsellor need to:

— Train existing service providers.
— Re-organise clinics to make better use of staff time.
— Recruit new staff and/or volunteers.

Lay volunteers are often trained in HIV counselling to fill the gaps in provision. The counsellor need to:

— Integrate the work of volunteers into that of other health workers.
— Consult them about ways to maintain their motivation.
— Give agreed rewards for the time and energy that they devote to a difficult task. In poor communities this should usually include material rewards.
— Design training courses that are tailored to meet the specific needs of the volunteers.
— Give frequent refresher training to update knowledge and skills.
— Provide practical items for example, notebooks, condoms, penis models, and leaflets.
— Respect and value the work of the volunteers and acknowledge their generosity to others.
— Arrange frequent meetings with volunteers to share achievements and problems, build support.

Counsellors need adequate training on all aspects of sexuality and STI/HIV counselling and supervised practice and support. They may not have covered sexuality, STI/HIV and gender relations adequately in previous training or may not have applied the training. Helping people to adopt safer sex practices may be more difficult than helping them to use contraception if it involves both partners in lifestyle changes and requires discussing intimate sexual practices. The counsellor need to spend time on relationship issues and enhancing clients' assertiveness and communication skills.

Topics need to cover basic information about STIs and HIV/AIDS, transmission routes, risk factors, possible and available interventions, pre-and post-HIV antibody test counselling and prevention counselling.

Counsellors may need new knowledge and skills, for example, on interventions to reduce HIV transmission from pregnant women to children. Health care workers may have had little training in HIV/AIDS care and may have similar attitudes to community members. Some issues, such as the benefits of replacement feeding, will contradict previous advice. Counsellors will need time and help to explore their own attitudes to sexual issues and how these may affect their counselling. This presents new challenges in being tolerant and talking about perhaps disapproved sexual practices.

Managers must acknowledge the importance of counselling on STI/HIV for their organisations, appreciate the staff who do this and allow them sufficient time to counsel. Many counsellors experience stress as a result of counselling on HIV. Managers need to provide regular support to minimise "burn out" and avoid losing valuable staff. Counsellors need to regularly change their tasks and have breaks from HIV counselling and also have access to counselling themselves.

Discussing HIV may raise personal anxieties for providers and may affect their ability to counsel others. Confidential counselling support and testing should be available. Language barriers may be a problem which confidential lay interpreters can help with. Knowledge of HIV/AIDS is changing fast. Counsellors need to keep uptodate to provide accurate information to clients, for example by updates from local HIV experts and the internet.

The counsellor need to change the organisation of his/her clinic to enhance privacy and client flows to enable young people and men to access the services. Some clinics have little time for counselling each client. There are a number of solutions to this problem:

i) *Move out of the clinic*: The clinic may not be the best place to counsel, particularly for clients for whom sexual activity is not approved. Community-based counsellors can meet people privately in a suitable place and provide more relaxed and accessible counselling.

ii) *Group information-giving*: Group information-giving can help to provide more people with knowledge but counsellors still need to check that clients understand the facts in relation to their own lives. Between 10 and 20 people in a group gives opportunities for discussion. The counsellor need to:

   a) Warn the group that you cannot guarantee confidentiality and it is safest to talk about issues in a general way rather than disclose personal information. This can happen later in the individual counselling sessions.

   b) Give the basic facts about HIV/AIDS, transmission routes, what the test can tell you, potential advantages and disadvantages of having the test and the process of counselling and testing. Give the information in a clear and interesting way that relates to people's lives.

   c) Ask the group if they have any questions and encourage discussion through the information giving.

iii) *Group counselling*: A group of about ten people who feel comfortable to talk together can discuss things in more depth. For example, single sex groups of a similar age and status, couples or families.

   a) Explain that people may wish to share their feelings and experiences but they must understand that confidentiality is not guaranteed in a group.

   b) Build rapport, explore issues around testing, options for risk reduction and coping mechanisms.

c) Encourage sharing of successful strategies for safer sex and coping and help people to gain more understanding of their options, the test and their own feelings.

iv) *HIV antibody counselling in antenatal clinics*: In some countries, HIV testing of all pregnant women is compulsory. All HIV testing should be voluntary, with women making an informed decision whether to be tested or not after counselling. Women attend antenatal clinics for the purpose of their own health and the health of their child. They are unprepared for HIV testing and often find it traumatic. They often have no signs or symptoms of STI or HIV and little knowledge about it. Women usually attend the antenatal clinic alone and this can make it very difficult to tell their partner about the test result. Providers and clients at the antenatal clinic may not be sufficiently aware of the level of confidentiality required in HIV testing. There is little privacy in many antenatal clinics. Therefore:

a) Counsel in privacy so that women feel comfortable to discuss sexual risk factors.

b) Provide a space where accompanying children can play with supervision.

c) Share confidential information about clients with providers to ensure that pregnant women get treatment and support and to reassure providers that they are not being put at risk.

d) HIV test counselling and ongoing support takes longer than the usual antenatal interview.

e) Giving pre-test information in groups can save time during counselling.

Ideally counsellors should provide services at times convenient to their clients. This may be easier if they are working outside the clinic, in the community. Counsellors need time to do good counselling on STI/HIV. Pre-HIV test counselling takes at least

30 minutes and post-test counselling after a positive result may take more than an hour and need to continue. Managers must recognise the time needed and plan accordingly.

Consider human, material and financial resources carefully and realistically before making decisions about what type of counselling to offer. Family planning and other local services may not have resources such as drugs needed to help clients who test HIV positive or have a STI. The counsellor need to tailor counselling to available resources, seek funding before starting or form partnerships with other organisations.

COUNSELLING AMONG PARTNERS

Partner counselling/notification involves the process of contacting sexual and/or injecting partners of an HIV-positive person in order to advise these partners that they may have been exposed to HIV and to encourage them to attend for HIV counselling, testing and, where applicable, treatment. The objectives of this kind of disclosure are to prevent HIV transmission to people who may be exposed either sexually or through needle-sharing and to improve care and support for people living with HIV or AIDS.

Partner counselling can be undertaken by the source client or patient him/herself, by the health care provider or through the combined efforts of both.

i) *Source referral:* HIV-positive people are encouraged to counsel partners concerning their possible exposure to HIV. This takes place without the direct involvement of health care providers. In this approach, the health care provider works with the HIV-positive person regarding the nature of the information to be passed on to their partner(s) and ways of doing it.

ii) *Provider referral:* An HIV-positive person gives the name(s) of his/her partner(s) to a health care provider who then confidentially counsels the partner(s) directly. In this approach, the health care provider does not disclose the name of the HIV-positive person to the partner, but only provides the information that the partner is likely to have been exposed to HIV infection. This is done with the consent of the source client or patient.

iii) *Conditional referral*: The health care provider of the source client or patient obtains the names of his/her sexual/drug-injecting partner(s), but allows the source client a period of time to counsel the partner(s) him/herself. If partners are not counselled within this time period, the health care provider counsels the partners, without naming the source patient or client concerned.

Partner counselling/notification has a long history as one possible aspect of the public health response to STIs other than HIV, such as syphilis and gonorrhoea. There is current debate whether, in the context of the transmission of HIV, the status and/or name of an HIV-positive person should be disclosed mandatorily to his or her sexual or drug-injecting partners. This is a particular concern in Africa and Asia where many women are being infected by their husbands or regular partners who do not reveal their HIV status or practise safe sex.

In the history of partner counselling, there are no clear data indicating that the mandatory counselling of partners is more effective in preventing transmission than the voluntary counselling of partners. It does appear that when people think that they will be forced to notify their partners, or that their status will be revealed without their consent, they choose not to attend for STI testing, counselling or other prevention and care services. This has been true in the case of syphilis and gonorrhoea even though, unlike HIV, these are curable and attract much less stigma and discrimination than HIV/AIDS.

It is even more likely that a policy of mandatory partner counselling will deter people from using HIV testing and counselling services, because there is greater incentive to fear testing and disclosure because of the serious stigma and discrimination surrounding HIV/AIDS. In fact, the reality is that, in many hospitals and clinics in low-income countries, disclosure of HIV status to sexual partners and others, such as family members, often takes place without consent. This happens because there are insufficient resources and personnel to store information in a way that respects privacy and/or because health care providers do not understand the professional duties of confidentiality and informed consent and their importance in the management of HIV/AIDS. This failure of health authorities to protect the privacy and autonomy of patients deters many people in these countries from seeking HIV counselling, testing and care.

It is not possible or practical to implement a large-scale scheme of mandatory partner counselling. It is virtually impossible to force people to test mandatorily for HIV, to retest periodically and to continue to inform partners, as would be necessary. Nor do people always know, or remember, the names of their sexual partners. Nor is it possible to force them to reveal them. Finally, it is very costly to train and employ staff to trace and counsel all those whose names are given.

However, it appears that mandatory partner counselling schemes are not necessary because voluntary partner counselling schemes can accomplish the critical goals. Voluntary partner counselling schemes can help to create a climate of confidence which will attract people to HIV testing and counselling services so that more people learn of their HIV status. Among those who do attend health care facilities and are faced with a decision whether to notify partners or not, it appears that most people agree to do so, on a voluntary basis, after counselling. In the context of a generally voluntary partner counselling programme, the small number of cases where persons refuse to notify their partners can be taken care of on an individual basis. Thus, for reasons of principle and because it is more feasible and capable of success, ethical partner counselling is encouraged by UNAIDS and WHO.

Ethical partner counselling is based on the informed consent of the source client or patient and, where possible, maintains the confidentiality of the source client or patient: that is, his/her name is not revealed to the partners being counselled. This will often be extremely difficult to maintain in the context of marital relationships, and requires the provision of counselling and support to both spouses to ensure the prospect of abuse and discrimination is minimised or eliminated.

Ethical partner counselling also takes into account the serious consequence of not counselling partners—possible HIV infection. This consequence requires an ethical weighing of the benefits and harm that are likely to occur if and when there is refusal on the part of an HIV-positive person to counsel partners.

UNAIDS and WHO encourage ethical partner counselling programmes which:

— employ serious counselling and persuasion towards counselling of partners;
— empower the health care provider, when the source client refuses to notify his/her partner, to make ethical decisions based on the potential harm and benefits to the parties, and decide whether to counsel the partner(s) without the consent of the source client;
— provide social and legal support for the source client and other relevant parties (spouses, partners, family members) to protect them from physical abuse, discrimination and stigma which may result from partner counselling.

UNAIDS and WHO advocate that there be greater exploration of concepts and practices concerning partner counselling which are culturally appropriate, ethically sound and effective in achieving prevention and care goals. One example is the concept of "shared confidentiality". The aim of shared confidentiality is to promote better support, care and prevention for individuals, families and communities affected by HIV/AIDS.

In communities where shared confidentiality has been a practice of community-based organisations, there has been an increase in community discussion of HIV/AIDS and a decrease in the stigma and discrimination surrounding HIV/AIDS. It has therefore helped to open up the HIV/AIDS epidemic in positive and supportive ways.

In Uganda and some other African countries, this notion of shared confidentiality has been developed by communities, NGOs and health care providers. A person affected by HIV is encouraged, and voluntarily chooses, to disclose his status to a range of people from whom he can get support.

There will be some cases where an HIV-positive person (source client) does not wish to, and may refuse to, notify his/her partner(s) or allow them to be counselled by the health care provider. Such refusal is most often due to a fear of rejection by partners and family, to fears of stigma and discrimination and/or to a fear of being blamed for the infection of others. It may also involve feelings of despair, remorse and guilt. Refusal to notify partners is very seldom due to a desire by the HIV-positive person to place another person deliberately at risk of HIV infection. For some, the consequences of their HIV status becoming known by their partners are severe. This is particularly the case for women who live in societies where women suffer social, economic and legal disadvantages because they are women. In such places, a woman is often blamed for her own infection, as well as for the infection of her husband/partner, even though it is likely that she was infected by him. The reaction to disclosing her status may also include physical violence and abandonment, in which she (and her children) may be thrown out of the home and given no economic or social support. Thus, women may have very valid reasons for fearing to disclose their status to husbands/partners.

Given the possible serious consequences of counselling partners (discrimination, abandonment, violence) and of not counselling partners (transmission of HIV infection), counsellors and health care workers must be trained to handle the difficult ethical decisions to be made. In each case, all the potential harm and benefits of counselling or not counselling partners should be weighed. In most cases, with counselling and with a demonstration of support, the HIV-positive person will agree to notify partners. Initial support may take the form of notification in the presence of the counsellor and/or in the presence of another family member who will provide support, and protection if necessary. Furthermore, there should be follow-up and referral to other support services to ensure that the couple or family can cope with the HIV among them.

In cases where the source client refuses to notify, following repeated efforts to persuade him/her to do so, and where the failure to notify creates a danger to a partner whose identity is known to the counsellor (in legal language "an identifiable risk to an identifiable third party"), the counsellor should be authorised to counsel the partner(s) without the consent of the source client.

In making this decision, the counsellor should ensure that the following factors are present.

— The HIV-positive person (source client) has been thoroughly counselled as to the need for partner notification/counselling.
— The counselling has failed to achieve the appropriate behavioural changes, including the practice of safe sex.
— The source client has refused to notify, or consent to the counselling, of his/her partner(s).
— A real risk of HIV transmission to the identifiable partner(s) exists.
— The source client is given reasonable advance notice of the intention to counsel by the health care worker.
— The identity of the source client is concealed from the partner(s) if this is possible in practice.
— Follow-up is provided to ensure support to those involved as necessary and to prevent violence, family disruption,

etc. Recommendations for encouraging ethical partner counselling.

To encourage ethical partner counselling, UNAIDS and WHO recommend the following:

— Develop national policies and public health legislation on partner counselling that protect the principles of confidentiality and informed consent, and provide for the limited and clearly defined circumstances under which partner counselling may take place without consent.

— Develop public health legislation that authorises health care providers to decide, on the basis of each individual case and ethical considerations, whether to counsel partners without the consent of the source client, under certain circumstances.

— Hold consultations among health care providers, government and affected communities about how to encourage ethical partner counselling and protect people who disclose their status through such counselling.

— Provide training and guidelines for health care providers and counsellors about how to protect confidentiality and informed consent in the context of partner counselling; how to encourage and assist voluntary partner counselling; how to make difficult ethical decisions in cases where there is refusal to counsel partners; and how to counsel partners in ways that harm is minimised and support is provided.

— Promote the establishment of professional ethical codes among health care and social service providers which require respect for confidentiality and informed consent in the context of partner counselling, and provide penalties for unethical conduct.

— Establish mechanisms for accountability and ways of making complaints in health care institutions and in communities when partners are counselled unethically by health care providers and other professionals.

— Support practical legal and social measures that address the vulnerability of people, particularly that of women, to stigma, physical violence and abandonment, including projects in the community which will assist in providing treatment, care, emotional support and protection from discrimination to those involved in partner counselling.
— Promote and support community projects about people's responsibility to protect themselves and others from HIV infection, particularly among men and boys.

COUNSELLING ON SEXUALITY

Sexuality is more than sexual behaviour and sexual intercourse. It includes social roles, personality, gender and sexual identity, biology, relationships, thoughts and feelings. It has changing significance for people in various stages of life. Sexuality is affected by age, gender, culture and sexual orientation. The expressions of sexuality are influenced by various factors including social, ethical, economic, spiritual, cultural and moral concerns.

People find it difficult to talk about sexuality and often only accept it when there are important reasons, such as protection from STI and HIV. People need to accept their own sexuality and communicate about it if they are to assess and reduce their risk of STI/HIV infection. Many clients would like to talk to their counsellor about their sexual relationships and intimacy. They may feel that this is the only person with whom they can share their feelings about sexual relationships and STI and HIV, without fear of discrimination.

The primary sexual attraction to the same, opposite or both sexes is termed as sexual orientation. Most societies find it hard to acknowledge and accept that homosexuality or bisexuality are a universal part of human sexuality. Many gays, lesbians or bisexuals neither experience nor desire a choice in their sexual orientation.

The sexual activities that people engage in are commonly called sexual behaviours. For example, a married man may have sex with men sometimes as well as his wife, but not identify himself as homosexual. Counselling aims to create a climate where all clients can express themselves without fear of discrimination. All people, whatever their HIV status, have sexual feelings and may need help to feel able to express those sexual feelings safely and happily.

Sexual pleasure depends on a variety of factors, including mood, where and why people have sex and what society feels is appropriate or not appropriate behaviour. Sexual satisfaction rises when there is more intimacy between the partners. Understanding and accepting our own sexual desires and those of our partner helps to build intimacy, as well as being close in non-sexual ways. Cultures differ greatly in how they view different types of relationships and sexual activities. Women are usually expected to follow stated rules more than men. Everyone has the right to pursue sexual happiness in their own way, but only where the happiness and health of others is not at risk. Forced sex is wrong. No one has the right to have sex with a partner if it degrades her or him to an impersonal object. Everyone has the right to say no to sex at any time. Sexual pleasure need not be limited to sexual intercourse.

Unsafe sex might be very pleasurable for clients. Discuss safer sex not only in terms of STI, HIV and pregnancy prevention, but also explore ways to make safer sex pleasurable. Enable clients to talk about same sex activities or more than one sexual partner even if they are married. Do not make any assumptions about their sexual behaviour. Be aware that sex may not be pleasurable or consensual for the client. Explore the relationship between gender relations and sexual pleasure.

It is important for counsellors to be aware of how gender roles and stereotypes influence sexual relationships. The inequity between men and women is reflected in sexual relationships, making both women and men vulnerable to STI/

HIV. There are often double standards on sexual activity. Women are expected to abstain from sex before marriage and be faithful in marriage, whilst men are 'allowed' or expected to be sexually active before marriage and to have sexual relations outside marriage.

In many societies, men are socialised to treat women as inferior in order to exercise power over them. Sexual acts do not always take place between two consenting adults, but involve domination of one person by another. Women and young people may not have the right to refuse sex if their partners or an older person asks for it. Disagreement over the use of preventive methods can lead to abusive situations. Men may feel that the prevention of unwanted pregnancies and even STI/HIV is a female concern. On the other hand, women who carry condoms or use contraceptives may be accused of promiscuity. This results in conflicts with men demanding unprotected sex but expecting women to protect themselves.

The sexual pleasure of men is often considered more important than that of women. Women are seen as providers and men as seekers of pleasure. Women may be accused of promiscuity if they ask for or obviously enjoy sex. Ignorance and lack of communication about sex may contribute to this problem. Men and women may not know about the importance of the clitoris for female pleasure or that women can have orgasms.

In some cultures, women are expected to have dry tight vaginas to please their partners. A sexually aroused woman is thought to be 'loose' or to have an STI. This practice puts them at risk of STI/HIV because the vagina wall easily tears and condoms are more likely to break. Some women undergo genital cutting, which can involve the removal of the clitoris and labia and closing of the opening to the vagina to a small hole. This makes sex painful and the trauma and bleeding put these women at higher risk of HIV. This practice is believed to preserve chastity and fidelity and gives men more control over women.

National laws may promote greater equity between men and women and positive sexual and reproductive health practices. These laws may be different from local norms related to culture, religion and class. The law may state that girls should not marry until they are 18 years old, but local culture promotes marrying girls after puberty to avoid premarital sex. Universal human rights and sexual and reproductive rights include the right to life and to bodily integrity and making our own decisions about sexual activity, marriage and having children.

How can counsellors help clients to empower themselves?

- Explore clients' opinions about gender inequalities in sexual life and challenge them.
- Help clients to understand the impact of gender inequality on their sexual lives and health and look for ways to change them.
- Collaborate with other organisations and groups in the area who are working to change gender norms, improve gender relations and make them more equitable. Explore the origins of harmful practices with male and female clients, and their advantages and disadvantages. Challenge clients to have a new perspective on them.
- Educate clients about laws and universal rights and seek ways to put them into practice.
- Counsel men and women separately, in couples, and in small single sex or mixed groups so that they understand the views and feelings of the opposite sex. Show images of responsible, caring and assertive men and women.
- Provide information on male and female sexuality and sexual response to enhance mutual sexual pleasure. Include this in local ways of socialising young men and women on their gender and sexual roles.
- Help clients to know their rights and practice assertiveness and negotiation skills through role-play.

HIV Transmission through Sexual Activities

HIV, the human immune-deficiency virus which causes AIDS (Acquired Immune deficiency Syndrome) is found in blood, semen, vaginal fluids and breastmilk. It can spread from one person to another through vaginal, anal or oral sex; blood transfusions; unsterilised needles or instruments and from mother to child during pregnancy, delivery or breast-feeding. HIV is transmitted more easily in a person with an STI. The prevention and prompt treatment of STI reduces HIV infection by nearly 60 per cent. There is currently no cure for HIV infection, although treatments are available to slow down the progress of HIV infection. HIV remains in the body after infection for life and may cause no signs and symptoms for many years. Signs and symptoms which may indicate HIV infection and AIDS include weight loss greater than 10 per cent of body weight; fever or diarrhoea for more than a month; persistent severe fatigue; cough for more than a month; itchy skin rashes, cold sores, shingles, thrush in the mouth and throat and swollen glands at two or more sites for more than three months. A positive HIV test is needed to diagnose HIV Infection or AIDS because other illnesses have similar signs and symptoms.

STIs are caused by viruses, bacteria or protozoa, which are sexually transmitted through vaginal, oral or anal intercourse. Only HIV and hepatitis may also be passed through blood transfusion and injections. Some STI, for example, herpes can be transmitted by kissing and body touching. STIs are a common problem in many parts of the world, even where HIV prevalence is low. Common STIs include gonorrhoea, chlamydia, syphilis, chancroid, herpes and pubic lice. Signs and symptoms of STI include: sores on the genitals, anus or lips, which may be painful or painless; unusual discharge from the penis or vagina, which may smell bad; burning pain on urination; itching, burning or soreness in genitals; lower abdominal pain; pain when having sex; unusual bleeding which is not a period and chills and fever.

STIs are serious because they can cause pelvic inflammatory disease, ectopic pregnancy, infertility, damage to unborn and new-born children, illness and death. STI's can progress more quickly and severely in people with HIV and may present slightly different symptoms. Some STI remain in the body without causing symptoms but can be transmitted to partners and unborn children and cause illness in the future. These include syphilis, hepatitis, herpes and chlamydia.

There are many different sexual activities that men and women, men and men or women and women may engage in to express their sexuality. Sexual intercourse involving penetration is only one of these, there are many more. When the counsellor help clients to assess their risk and make a risk reduction plan, he needs to help them to talk about what activities they engage in. In this way, the clients will be aware of the risk level of all potential activities and have many pleasurable possibilities to consider. The list of activities in the boxes below is not complete—add others that he know about and ask the clients if they have any others.

Research has shown that it is possible to transmit HIV through oral sex, but cases where this has happened are rare. As far as we know receiving oral sex appears safer than giving oral sex. The risk of HIV transmission through oral sex is greater if the person or partner has an untreated STI such as gonorrhoea or syphilis. Untreated STIs are easily transmitted through oral sex.

Oral sex on a woman. This is risky during a menstrual period or when the person doing the oral sex has bleeding gums, mouth ulcers or open sores in the mouth or throat. Oral sex on a woman with HIV is less risky than oral sex with a man who has HIV. Barriers such as 'dental dams' can be used during oral sex with a woman.

Oral sex on a man. This is safer if the man wears a condom. It is risky without condoms if the person doing the oral sex has bleeding gums, mouth ulcers or any open sores.

Counsellors need to be aware of the most common physical and emotional problems clients may have with sex. They have to reflect together on giving and receiving sexual pleasure by exploring the client's personal experiences with sexual pleasure. Explain how their own and their partner's body functions. Discuss personal and social contexts for sex and factors like place, time, and frequency. Explore the factors that affect the clients' sexual pleasure.

COUNSELLING ON SAFER SEX, STI AND HIV

Counselling on safer sex, STI and HIV helps clients to assess their own risks of HIV infection and STI in the past, now and in the future and to make a plan to reduce risks. It aims:

i) To helps clients, whatever their HIV status, re-think their sexual lives and find ways to enjoy safer sex.
ii) To help clients to feel positive about male/female condom use.
iii) To identify clients who have a Reproductive Tract Infection (RTI) or STI so that they can receive prompt treatment and prevent (further) infection in partners.
iv) To help clients to take RTI/STI treatment correctly.
v) To help clients with STI to inform all their partners of the need to go for check up and treatment.

The counsellor has to find his own ways to introduce the topic of STI and HIV in a counselling session. If clients come and express concerns about HIV or STI, affirm their sense of responsibility and decision to take action. Assure them of confidentiality. Each client will have their particular needs, so the counsellor has to give all clients an opportunity to discuss and get help on any aspect of their sexual lives.

Many people wish to protect their fertility and have healthy children and one of the ways the counsellor can help clients do this is to protect themselves from STI/HIV. He may find it

Table 1. Safe and Unsafe Sex

Safe Sex	Safer Sex	Unsafe Sex
These are sexual activities (SA) with no risk of HIV transmission. - All SA between two uninfected people are safe. - All SA that do not and could not involve semen, vaginal fluids or blood going from one person into another are safe. These include: - Massage - Hugging - Solo masturbation - Body to body rubbing (not genitals) - Sex talk, sexy dancing - Sharing sexual fantasies - Body kissing - Showering together - Using sex toys without sharing them.	*These are sexual activities (SA) with a low risk of STI and HIV transmission.* - SA involving a person with HIV infection where there is no semen, vaginal fluid or blood going from one person into another. - Activities that are theoretically safe at this time and are not known to have been a route for infection. *These include:* - Masturbation of each other if there are no cuts on the hands and people don't touch their own genitals afterwards. - Open mouth kissing if both partners have no bleeding gums or cuts in the mouth. - Vaginal intercourse with a condom. - Gentle anal intercourse with a condom and plenty of waterbased lubricant.	*These are high-risk sexual activities.* - Any practice with a person who might have HIV infection that allows blood, semen or vaginal fluids inside the body through the mucous membranes of the mouth, vagina, penis or anus or through broken skin. *These include:* - Vaginal and anal intercourse without a condom - Any type of blood contact, including menstrual blood, semen or vaginal fluid entering breaks in the skin. - Sharing sex toys without cleaning them between partners - Any type of sex that damages the delicate tissues in the vagina, head of penis or rectum. For example, dry sex, rough sex, abrasive substances in vagina.

easier to begin to talk about the risk of STI/HIV when he is helping the clients to choose a contraceptive method. He could then begin a more in depth exploration of their risk and options for reducing it. If the client says nothing about HIV in a family planning counselling session, the counsellor might say something like:

"There is a lot of concern these days about HIV and AIDS. The counsellor can give all the clients an opportunity to discuss this issue with the counsellor so that they can think about their own lives and take any necessary action to stay safe. Would you like to do this?" If clients do not wish to talk about STI or HIV, the counsellor can to ensure that they are aware of the potential risk of STI and HIV and what they can do to reduce those risks. Encourage the clients to tell about any genital signs or symptoms that concern them.

Women are often too embarrassed to talk about genital problems. The counsellor need to ask: "Do you have any problems in your private parts that you would like to talk to me about? For example, vaginal discharge?" "Do you have any worries about illnesses passed through sex that you would like to talk to me about?" Offer visual screening for signs and symptoms of STI. Explain that some women do not show any signs or symptoms of STI but the germs can still be damaging their organs. Offer the client screening tests and explain the test procedure.

Helping to Assess the risk of STI and HIV

The counsellor can help the client to assess the risk of STI and HIV. Begin with sharing knowledge about how STI/HIV is transmitted and then exploring the possibility of transmission in clients' lives. Help them to reflect on their past and present sexual and drug-using behaviour and whether this may have put them at risk of STI and HIV infection. They also need to think about their medical history and whether they might be at risk from blood transfusions.

Help clients to talk about all their sexual activities and partners. Do not make any assumptions about clients' sexual activity nor the activity of their sexual partners. The client may have or have had partners of the same sex or the opposite sex now or in the past. A married person may have relationships outside marriage or their partner may have such relationships. An adolescent may be abused at home.

Provide information on the level of risk of different sexual activities. Probe about other possible activities that the client may not have thought significant or may not like to mention. Discuss each of their concerns in detail, learning about their understanding of HIV and adding information as needed. When all their concerns have covered, ask about any risk factors that they have not mentioned. Summarise the main points and ask how the client feels about their likely risk. Share the assessment of their likely risk. Move on to make a risk reduction plan or talk about the HIV test if appropriate.

Helping to Reduce the Risk of STI/HIV Infection

Options for safer sex include:

i) abstinence from penetrative sex.
ii) uninfected partners being faithful to each other.
iii) using condoms every time you have sexual intercourse.

Different options may suit people at different times of their lives. The counsellor can help the clients to explore the three options above. Explain that they can make a choice that suits them now and change it as their circumstances or preferences change. Clients, whether living with HIV or not may have to rethink their sexual relationships. Support clients at risk in finding other ways than intercourse to express their sexual feelings if condoms are not available or they don't feel able to use them. Recap on all the sexual activities with the client and their level of risk. Give the client information on other activities that they might enjoy as appropriate and on how to make preferred activities safer.

Explore with the client the good and bad points of each choice in terms of level of HIV (and pregnancy) prevention, enhancing relationships, intimacy and pleasure, partner's preference, other consequences, practicality and feelings. Help clients to think about potential results of each choice. Help clients to come to their own decision. They may need more time to think about the options and discuss them with others. Women may put themselves at risk of abuse if they speak to their partners about condoms or fidelity without careful thought and preparation.

When clients have expressed a preference, help them to explore in more detail to check on whether it is a good choice and to think about how to put their intentions into practice. Help the client to gain any skills needed to put their plan into action, for example, how to use condoms and talk to their partner.

Helping clients to abstain from sex: Abstinence means a person does not engage in vaginal or anal sexual intercourse. Some people believe that abstinence means no sexual activity of any kind, others that people who are abstaining may still engage in non-penetrative sexual activities. Some people think that it is easier to abstain if they do not engage in any sexual activity at all because they may find it difficult to stop without intercourse.

Abstinence may be a good choice for young people who are in unequal power relationships or feel unready to have sex, people who do not have a faithful partner and/or who value sex for a special relationship or marriage or those who are not able to have sex because of separation or illness. People may say that they intend to give up sex because of HIV, but it is important that they plan different ways to protect themselves in case they change their minds.

Helping clients to enjoy sexual pleasure without intercourse: People who are abstaining may still express their sexual feelings by the non-penetrative sexual activities. Women and men's sexuality differs and some women may actually get more pleasure from sexual activities other than intercourse. The dominance of men has tended to focus sex on intercourse and many people feel that this is the 'real' sex, the sex that results in conception. Others think that non-penetrative sexual activities are enjoyable and valid and do not feel that intercourse is essential for expressing their sexuality. In some cultures young people are taught how to express themselves sexually without intercourse. In others, young people learn by themselves or from each other how to please each other without intercourse. This sexual play can be safe and enjoyable for both people.

The main risk is that the couple become so excited that they are not able to stop and go on to have unprotected intercourse. Unless there is trust and commitment, the man might force the woman to have intercourse with the excuse that he is unable to stop. Some people may enjoy sex without intercourse for a long period of time. For others, one or both partners may become very frustrated and tense and this can cause conflicts in the whole relationship.

The counsellor can help the clients to explore all potential safe and safer sexual activities and to find strategies for introducing them in their relationships if necessary and reducing the risk of unprotected intercourse. He can help people to move from sex without intercourse to sex with condoms or to move towards VCT and a stable relationship, if the choice to enjoy sexual pleasure without intercourse is not working well for the client.

Helping clients to stay with uninfected partners who only stay with them: This choice is important in reducing HIV infection, particularly where HIV transmission rates are low or condoms are not available, affordable or acceptable. Clients and their partners can only know that they are both uninfected if they have an HIV test and practice safer sex from then on. Or if they became sexual partners as virgins and then had no other sexual partners, blood transfusions or unsterilised injections since then.

HIV can stay in the body for 10 or more years without symptoms so people who had unprotected sex before marriage may be HIV positive even though they have not had any other partners after marriage. In many cultures, men and sometimes women have several sexual partners before they marry.

HIV testing and discussions about possible HIV infection in stable relationships are difficult because they can imply a lack of trust and fidelity. Many couples stop using condoms after they have been together for six months or so because they now 'trust' each other. They may wish to conceive a child. However, the decision to practice safe sex has nothing to do with trust because without an HIV test, no-one who has been sexually active can know whether they are infected or not.

Married people may have secret sexual relations outside marriage and never tell their partner. Partners may be unaware of risk. Married people may use condoms with outside partners to protect themselves and their family from infection without telling their spouses. This strategy does not allow the spouse to make an informed decision on the level of risk they are willing to live with because condoms do not provide 100 per cent protection.

Counsellors often find it difficult to counsel married women on HIV because it requires them to acknowledge that their spouses might have outside partners and then talk to them about it. If the woman decides not to talk to her partner, she may become anxious and cease to enjoy sexual relations. If she does talk to him, it may result in rejection, abuse or violence.

Helping clients to use condoms: The counsellor can give a description of the use of condoms. A brief discussion about the use of male and female condoms are given below.

i) *Use of male condom*: A man can use a thin rubber sock called a condom. The man or woman unrolls the condom onto his erect penis before sex starts. The condom prevents the man's sperm from getting inside the woman, so they cannot join with the egg. This prevents pregnancy.

Condoms also protect against STI/HIV infection because the germs that cause these infections cannot get through the condom from the man to the woman, the woman to the man, or the man to the man. After ejaculation, before the penis gets soft, the man withdraws and carefully removes the condom. He takes care not to spill any sperm on the woman's genitals. Condoms are very effective if they are used correctly and consistently at every act of intercourse. The condom should be put on before any genital contact. They are even more effective against pregnancy if a spermicide like Neo-sampoon is used with them. If people do not use them all the time, they are much less effective than other methods against pregnancy. However, they are the only method that currently protects against STI including HIV. It is better to use condoms sometimes than not at all.

Condoms have no effects on the body except in about 8 per cent of people who are allergic to rubber. They allow the man to take some responsibility for family planning. It is important to store condoms in a cool, dry place out of sunlight. Condoms are a good choice for people who want to have dual protection from pregnancy and STI/HIV. They are also a good choice for clients who have sex infrequently or do not want drugs or devices affecting their reproductive system.

Condoms are a first choice method for breast-feeding mothers because they have no effect on breast milk production and protect mother and baby from STI and HIV infection through breast milk. They are good in cultures where people believe that semen will poison breastmilk because the condom prevents the semen from reaching the breast-milk. Condoms are the best choice for young people because they protect against STI/HIV. This protects their future fertility and life and prevents pregnancy. However, young people need to be motivated and helped to use them regularly and correctly. Many couples find they enjoy sex more with condoms because they do not have to worry about pregnancy and STI/HIV. Also, condoms can help prevent premature ejaculation.

Counsellors should follow the steps given below to help the client to use male condoms in a safe manner:

— Ask whether the client has any experience of using condoms. If they do, ask them about their experiences, any problems they faced, how condoms affected their sexual life, any worries they have about them and what they think about using them again.

— Provide information as needed. Demonstrate how to put on a condom.

— If the client has no experience of using condoms, ask what they have heard about them, how they feel about them and what barriers they might have to using them.

— When you have understood the client's concerns about condoms, explore how they might be solved. Always be honest about the problems that can arise with condoms, but also be positive and say that many people use them happily.

Some ways to help clients with worries about condoms are given below.

Ways to reduce the risk of breakage:

— Avoid dry sex and do not put powders into the vagina. If the woman is dry, use spermicide foam or water-based jelly.

— Do not use Vaseline or any oil on the condom, it will spoil the rubber.

— Do not use condoms that are more that five years older than the date of manufacture on the packet. If the condoms have been kept in a warm place they will last for less time than this.

How to minimise the risk if a condom does break:

— Use a spermicide as a double layer of protection;

— Stop sex at once if either of you feel the condom break and pull out. If the man has not ejaculated the risks are low. Put spermicide into the vagina.

— Go to the nearest clinic for emergency contraception as soon as possible, but at least within 72 hours of the breakage.

ii) *Use of female condom:* The female condom is a sock made of plastic with a ring at each end. It works in the same way as the male condom by stopping sperm getting into the vagina during sex. The female condom protects against pregnancy, STI and HIV in the same way as the male condom. It is about 98 per cent reliable if used correctly every time. Female condoms are popular in some places. Women may find it easier to negotiate or insist on the use of the female condom than the male condom. Men and women may find them more comfortable than male condoms because they are looser. They may be seen as 'respectable' for married couples, perhaps because they are new.

To insert the condom: Wash your hands. Rub the condom to spread the lubricant. Hold the ring of the closed end. Squeeze the ring. Put the condom into the vagina as far as it will go. The ring should be at the end of the vagina. Push the condom up the vagina, leaving the other ring outside the body. Make sure that the condom is not twisted. Make sure that the outer ring is lying on the vulva. During sex, ensure the penis is inside the condom and not between the wall of the vagina and the condom. To remove, squeeze and twist the outer ring, pull out, wrap carefully and put in latrine or a place where children cannot find it. For extra moisture and comfort use saliva, spermicide or an oil-based lubricant inside the condom.

Disposal of condoms: Explain the dangers of throwing condoms anywhere. Ask how the client will be able to dispose of the condoms. What might make it difficult? Try to find a solution to any barriers to disposal. Maybe the client could dig a latrine or wrap it in paper or leaves until he/she reaches one.

Helping clients whose partners refuse to use condoms: A man or a woman might refuse to use condoms for a number of reasons.

— Explore with the client why they think their partner does not want to use condoms. Empathise and think about what might help them to try condoms. If it is helpful, role-play the situation with you as the client and the client playing his or her partner. This can help them to understand their partner better.

— For many people, skin to skin contact and the intimacy between people during sex is very highly valued both physically and spiritually. It is not easy for people to change these deeply held values.

— Some men have difficulty getting or maintaining an erection using a condom. Couples may get used to the condom in time and forget that they are using it. Help the client to focus on pleasuring the body. If it is helpful, try to counsel both partners, either together or separately.

Negotiation techniques: Negotiation is a discussion with another person, in order to reach a mutual agreement on a given issue. Acquiring skills in negotiating for safer sex is therefore very important. Ways to help negotiation to go well:

— Ensure that the environment and surroundings are comfortable, private and with no interruptions or distractions

— Give both of you enough time, whenever appropriate, to focus on the discussion. Avoid awkward situations, for example after a quarrel.

— Tell your partner that you want to discuss something important in advance and agree a time and place to allow you both time to prepare for the discussion.

— Be confident and say clearly what you know, feel and think without hurting your partner. Be sure of your facts and committed to change. Say clearly what you would like and do not be afraid of losing or offending your partner. Be assertive rather than attacking or pleading. Don't blame him or her.
— Encourage your partner to make the first contribution to the discussion and give him or her time to speak and think. This will help you to see how he or she is feeling about the issue and it will help you to relax.
— Be ready to listen to your partner with an open mind. Don't assume you know how he or she thinks and feels.
— Try to have a positive attitude. Stay calm and try to reach an agreement on each point as you go along; this helps to build a positive atmosphere.
— Try to talk your partner into agreement in a loving way rather than threatening or begging.
— You might need to ask for help and support from a very close relative or a friend and ask him or her to talk to your partner on the issue in your absence.

The most important point of all is that, in order to succeed in negotiating for safer sex, the client must know the facts about HIV and AIDS and about safer sex options.

Counselling Client with an STI Diagnosis

In counselling client with an STI siagnosis the counsellor should follow the steps given below.

i) Affirm the client and assure her or him of confidentiality.
ii) Encourage the client to tell you about any signs and symptoms, recent sexual interactions, fears and what they have already done to try to solve the problem.
iii) Explain that the examination or test showed that they have an infection in their genitals passed through sexual

intercourse. Explain and answer the client's questions about it.

iv) Explain that STIs can have serious consequences if they are not treated as quickly as possible. Explain the potential consequences of the client's particular STIs if they are not treated.

v) Explain that most STIs are curable if they are treated early with a complete course of the correct drugs. Explain about the prognosis for the clients STI. Stress the importance of taking the full course of correct drugs. Too little of the correct drug may make the infection difficult to cure next time. Wrong drugs or local treatments may not kill all the pathogens or cure the infection.

vi) If necessary, refer the client to the best local facility for STI treatment and discuss any barriers he has to seeking treatment there. If he has concerns about issues such as travel, costs, attitudes of providers and confidentiality, look for ways to work with the service providers to improve the quality or get an exemption.

vii) Explain what will happen at the health unit, when it opens and what the nurse will need to know and do.

viii) Explain that clients need to tell all their sexual partners about the infection so that they get treatment. If women have no symptoms and are not told and treated, they may become very ill or infertile and they are at higher risk of HIV. Also, partners can re-infect each other every time they have sex if they are not both treated.

ix) Generally it is difficult for women to tell men about STI infection because of gender inequality and men often do not wish to tell their partners. This is a serious problem, which you can help to solve in collaboration with community programmes.

x) Explore the best way for clients to tell their partners about the infection. Think about when, where, who and how. If it helps, role-play the best approach and timing. Ask how the partner might react to the news and what the client could do to minimise risk of rejection, conflict or abuse.

xi) If clients are anxious about telling their partners or are not able to do so, explore alternatives with them. Take great care not to push them into a potentially dangerous situation.

Partners may refuse to come for an STI test and/or treatment, especially if they do not have symptoms. They may wish to go to a different facility and/or take treatment without counselling or a test. Clients may refuse to tell their partners because they blame them or they want to keep their outside relationships secret. Some people lie to their stable partners about the nature of an STI. This may prevent quarrels but everyone has a right to information about their risk of STI/HIV. Understanding of the risks of infertility and damage to babies can motivate people to seek STI treatment promptly and to inform their partners. Understanding the increased risk of HIV and its impact on both clients and families can motivate a change of behaviour.

Group counselling for men can help to change attitudes. Both partners should abstain from sex until they are completely cured. If they are unable to do this, they should use condoms each time they have sex. Explain that STIs increase the risk of HIV. Stress the importance of prevention of STI and ask if clients wish to consider taking an HIV test.

If the client is in an ongoing relationship, STIs frequently result in conflicts because they imply that one or both parties have had a relationship outside. Women are often blamed, punished and rejected more than men, although their stable partner often infects them. Ask the client how she or he is feeling. Give her or him time to express their feelings about the situation.

While counselling a couple, give them a chance to say how they feel to each other while the other person really listens. Give positive examples of couples who have been in this situation and come through it and are still together. Help the couple to really listen and talk to each other about their thoughts and feelings to increase their understanding. Help them to talk about what they like sexually and what they can both do to avoid this problem in future. In this way, the counsellor have an opportunity to help the couple to talk more openly about what is going on in their sexual lives. Although this can be painful, it may finally help the relationship. While counselling one person, use role-play to practice communication.

Clients may need more support in talking to their partners, accessing and taking the correct treatment, and changing their own behaviour or that of their partners so they are not infected again. Arrange the next meeting to see whether they are cured and how their relationship is going. Find out whether they have been to the health unit, what medicine they are taking and whether the signs and symptoms have gone.

Counselling before HIV Antibody Testing

Counselling before HIV antibody testing aims to help the client to freely make an informed choice on whether or not to take the HIV antibody test on the basis of full and accurate information on the potential benefits and costs in their lives. The counsellor should find out what clients know about the HIV antibody test. Explain how the HIV antibody test works, the window period and the meaning of a positive, negative and uncertain result. Help clients to explore the advantages and disadvantages of taking the test in their own lives. Table 1 gives some ideas on this.

Never persuade or pressure clients to have an HIV antibody test. For any individual, the disadvantages of doing this may outweigh the advantages, particularly if testing facilities are poor or they are not in a powerful position in the family.

Some clients may decide to have a test, but then think more about the advantages and disadvantages when they go home and discuss it with others. They may then decide not to come for the results. These clients are not 'drop-outs' – this is part of the informed choice process. If the client decides to have the test, continue with the next steps. If the client decides not to have the test, help them to summarise their risk reduction plan and support them in their action. Encourage them to visit again at any time for further counselling.

Table 2
Advantages and disadvantages of HIV antibody test

Advantages	*Disadvantages*
The test can: Motivate people to reduce their risk of HIV infection and the risk of infecting others. Enable couples to enjoy any kind of sexual activity without condoms if both partners are negative and stay only with each other. Enable couples to make an informed decision on whether to have children or not. Help parents to take action to reduce the risk of mother to child transmission. Help health workers to provide the best treatment to patients with HIV. Help people to join a support group. Stop people worrying and help them to take positive action whatever the result. Help to normalise HIV and reduce stigma if more people take the HIV test and are open about their status.	Rarely people may get a false positive or negative result, then they may suffer distress and severe consequences unnecessarily. Or they may worsen their own health or infect others unknowingly. People may react badly to a positive result. They may drink too much or have unsafe sex. They may become depressed and suicidal. People with a positive result may lose their marriage, children, home and job if others get to hear about it. Women are very vulnerable, they may be isolated, beaten and stigmatised, with severe long-term effects on their well-being and family lives. People with a negative result may be so relieved that they have more risky sex, thinking that they are immune. If a person with a positive result does not have the power to do anything about it, they may feel more anxious and unhappy after the test.

Obtaining consent for HIV testing: Explain that the test is voluntary; no-one is forced to have it. Ensure that the clients understand and have considered the implications of having the test. If they decide to have the test, ask them to state specifically that they wish to have the test and do not feel under any pressure from anyone to do so. Set up procedures to ensure that informed consent is given.

Cost of test: Tell the client the cost of having the test if they have to pay for it. Ask if this presents any problems for them. Try to set up an exemption scheme for those who cannot afford the test. Explain the testing options available and explain how the test will be done and when the results will be ready. Remind them about the window period, the need to avoid exposure to HIV before the test and the meaning of the results. Help clients to prepare for a positive or negative result. This can help clients to respond better to the results and take positive actions as early as possible. It helps the counsellor to support them in a more informed way.

Explore past anxiety, depression and tendency to self harm or alcohol and drug abuse. Explain that couples may have different HIV test results. One partner may be positive and the other negative. This is called a discordant couple. This can happen because one person was exposed to HIV outside this relationship and has not infected the other person because of condom use, immunity or low exposure of the partner.

It is important that clients think about how they will cope when they get the test results and who will support them. It is very important that they do not tell anyone without thinking about it carefully because of stigma. Ask:

— How do you cope with problems in your life – who helps you, what makes you feel strong and able to cope, do you have activities like religion which give you courage?
— Could you tell me about your family situation?
— Do you belong to any networks of friends, community support groups, clubs, religious or other groups that support you?

— Who do you think would help you if the test result was positive? Or negative?
— Did you tell anyone that you were thinking of having an HIV antibody test? Why that person?
— Who would you tell about the test results.

Pressure may be put on people to have an HIV antibody test by partners, family, religious body, workplace or visa departments. Some interventions are only accessible to people who have agreed to have an HIV antibody test. Putting pressure on someone in any way to have an HIV antibody test is a violation of human rights and unethical. Counsellors should explain this and explore alternatives if clients wish.

Premarital HIV Counselling

It is common in some places for couples to have an HIV test before marriage. Sometimes one or both of them decide to do this themselves, sometimes the church or their families demand it. Some religious bodies refuse to marry people if one or both have HIV infection. This is a violation of human rights. If couples or individuals are obliged to have a test before marriage, the testing is no longer voluntary and there is no informed consent.

Pre-marital counselling and testing can help couples to:

— Make an informed decision about whether to get married.
— Talk about their sexual life together.
— Make informed decisions about safer sex and the need for condom use.
— Motivate couples to practice safer sex from now on.
— Make informed decisions about having children.

A positive test result can lead to rejection and distress, particularly if one person tests positive. However, some couples stay together, support each other and grow in their love. If the test is not voluntary, explain that testing should be voluntary and they have a right to give informed consent. If they wish, explore their possible risk of infection, the pros and cons of the test and what might happen if one or other or both had a positive or negative result. Talk through options with them, for example, to marry in a different way that does not demand a test or to discuss it further with family and partners. Help them to reduce their risk of HIV infection in their marriage. If they decide to take the test, help them to prepare for it.

An HIV positive result means that the test has detected antibodies to HIV in the blood. It does not mean that the person has AIDS or that they will soon die. If people with a positive result are healthy, they have HIV infection and may live for many years. If people with a positive result have illnesses related to HIV infection, they may have AIDS and can be helped with treatment and care.

Rarely some HIV tests give a false positive result. The test should be repeated and confirmed if possible with Western Blot before disclosing the positive result to clients. An HIV negative result means that the test did not detect any antibodies to HIV in the blood. If the person has not been exposed to HIV within the past three-music months, they are most likely not infected with HIV. If they have been exposed to HIV in the past three-six months, they may not yet have made antibodies. They may still be infected. In this case, the person needs to have another test in three months time to know their HIV status.

An uncertain result means that the test did not clearly show whether antibodies were present or not. A person may be in a sero-conversion phase and will require another test. It is best to have the same counsellor doing pre-test and post-test counselling because they have a stronger partnership and trust, the counsellor is familiar with the client's situation and they can more easily refer back to the plans made by the client in pre-test counselling.

There is a wide range of possible client reactions to a positive test result, ranging from anger, resignation, bargaining, depression to severe shock and disbelief. Some clients assume they will immediately become ill and die. Clients often show strong emotions, which many of us are not used to coping with, especially in a constrained work situation. The client may speak of suicide, threaten others, be angry with the counsellor or be unable to cope.

Clients' psychological responses depend on a number of factors including history and personality, social support and coping mechanisms and quality of pre-test counselling. If the client has not had good pre-test counselling, the counsellor should spend more time explaining things to them after the test and helping them to make plans.

Understanding the result

— Ask clients how they have been feeling since they had the blood drawn and congratulate them for returning or waiting to hear their test results.

— Ask clients if they have any questions or if they want to talk over anything before you give them their results. Most clients will want to hear their test result as soon as possible.

— When clients are ready, give the test result in a neutral voice and wait for the client to respond before proceeding.

For a positive test result, say: Your test result was positive; that means that you are infected with HIV'. For a negative test result say: 'Your test result was negative; that means we did not detect any antibodies for HIV'. Find language which makes the meaning of the test clear to clients. If they are not from a scientific background explain HIV and antibodies in a local way. Ask clients what they understand by the test result. Talk it over until they understand. Ask if they have any other questions about the result.

Expressing emotions: Ask the clients how they are feeling. Encourage them to express their emotions freely and do not rush them or try to stop them.

Making a plan: When clients are clear about the meaning of the result and have expressed their initial feelings, they may be ready to talk about what to do next and make an immediate plan. Ask "What are you planning to do when you leave here today?" If clients made a plan in pre-test counselling, they need to talk through it again in detail because they may feel very differently now they know their results. The plan might include telling their partner, modifying their risk reduction plan or seeking medical help. Clients who are HIV positive are likely to need more than one counselling session to come to terms with their results and make and carry out their plan.

Counselling HIV Positive Clients

Telling clients that they have HIV infection is distressing and difficult for counsellor and client. If the client does not have AIDS, explain the difference between HIV and AIDS again and say that many people remain healthy for a long period of time with HIV infection.

Psychological support: The counsellor have a very important role in providing psychological support to clients and helping them to access support systems at home.

- — Identify and explore clients' feelings.
- — Ask questions like "would you like to tell me more".
- — Let clients know that their feelings are natural and that they are likely to change after the initial shock of learning the test result
- — Talk over again the questions you discussed during the pre-counselling session.
- — Explore how clients were able to deal with other difficult situations in the past.
- — Identify sources of support available to the client, for example, family, friends, partner, church and clubs. Give the client any additional information about local sources of support, such as groups for People living with HIV or

AIDS (PLWHA), church members and counselling organisations.

— Explore the client's ability to cope and ways of coping. These might include song, prayer, long walks, spending time with family and friends or joining a support group.

— If the client expresses any suicidal thoughts or ideas, take them seriously, even if the test is anonymous and confidential. Make sure that they have support before you see them next time.

— Assess the client's medical, preventive, and psychological support needs and discuss access to existing services.

Making a plan:

— Ask the client what they are planning to do when they leave the session and, if necessary, remind them of the plan they made in the pre-test session for what they would do if their result was positive. Talk through the plan with them.

— Assess the client's social support and plans for partner notification.

— Help the client to establish a plan for continuing medical, social and psychological support.

— Help clients to identify possible actions that may help resolve or ease their problems.

— Identify with clients tasks that they feel able to accomplish with the counsellor's support.

— Set up a follow-up session or refer as appropriate

Making a risk reduction plan. Discuss again the client's risk for transmitting HIV infection to others. Reinforce the message about prevention of HIV transmission and safer sex. Many clients who test HIV positive are not concerned about safer sex in the first post-test counselling session. However, they still need to protect their partners from infection and themselves from re-infection. Discuss clients' responsibility to ensure that their partners are notified and counselled about their exposure to HIV. If they feel unable to do this, discuss how they can reduce the risk of infecting their partners. If the client agrees, help with a plan to contact the partners. Remind clients of their risk reduction plan.

Practising protected sex is often easier if both partners know their HIV status. If they are both positive, they can protect each other from re-infection with HIV and with other STIs. This will help to maintain their immunity. If one person is negative and the other positive (a discordant couple) they can protect each other and help the uninfected person to stay negative.

Counselling over time can help individual clients to tell their sexual partners about their status. If a woman has an HIV positive test result and she does not know the sero-status of her partner, she needs to find ways to protect herself and him from infection. If she suspects that he infected her and is therefore positive himself, she still needs to protect the two of them from re-infection, because this can speed up the progression of the infection. The same thing applies if the man is positive but the wife has not had a test. Discuss the possibility of encouraging sexual partners to have an HIV antibody test. An HIV positive test result can result in sexual problems for either partner. The person may feel too afraid of infecting their partner to engage in sex at all. When someone discovers that they are infected with HIV, they face a difficult decision about whether to tell anyone.

Disclosure: Disclosure is a process and not an event. It is a major decision that can have consequences for the person living with HIV and those around him or her. It is important that people do not rush into disclosure, but think it through carefully and plan ahead. Planning allows the client to imagine what may happen when he or she tells different people about their status and how they will control it. Steps towards disclosure include:

— Help the client to take time to think things through. Never judge people or put any pressure on them to tell others.

Protect them from pressure from others and make sure that they want to tell people.

— Help clients to realise that it may be easier to tell one or two trusted people at first. Discuss sexual partners and children who need protection from HIV if appropriate.

— Help clients to understand what might happen if they tell inappropriate people or groups about their status.

— Help clients to make a plan for telling others. This should cover who they will tell first and later, how and where they will tell them, how much they will say and preparations.

— Discuss what different peoples' reactions might be immediately and afterwards. Prepare clients for shocked or hostile reactions. These are common but usually turn to acceptance with time. They will need to assess how much the person understands about HIV and AIDS. This will help them to decide what they need to tell the person and how to tell it so that it is less traumatic for both of them.

— Role-play telling different people with the client or using an 'empty chair' to represent the person. Invite the client to role-play the person being told so that they can empathise with the person and imagine the best way to go about it. The role-plays also act as a rehearsal and give the client confidence.

— Help the client to feel strong enough to allow others to express their feelings and concerns after they have been told.

Making decisions about having children

— Help HIV positive clients to decide what to do about having children. If they decide to postpone or not have children, help them decide which contraceptive to use.

— If clients want to conceive or are pregnant, discuss how anti-retrovirals (ARV), if available, could help them to reduce the risk of infection in the baby and slow their own infection.

— Pregnant women might wish to discuss the possibility of termination if it is legal at the number of months of the pregnancy.

Helping clients with HIV infection to live positively

— Explain that many people with HIV infection have learned to live positively and this has helped them to stay well and productive for a longer time.

— Living positively means living as normally as possible and looking after your health, psychological and other needs.

— Discuss the following ideas with clients and help them to make plans for living as positively as possible.

- Try to eat meals containing energy foods such as cereals and tubers; oil and butter; body-building foods such as beans, nuts, seeds, fish, meat, eggs and milk; and fruits and vegetables to provide vitamins and minerals.
- Continue with work as long as you feel able to.
- Take enough rest.
- Try to stop smoking and only drink alcohol in moderation.
- Find ways to reduce stress.
- Seek spiritual support.
- Seek treatment for infections promptly.
- Explore the possibility of having anti-retroviral (ARV) treatment to slow down the infection with the client.

— Preparing for the future can help people to feel more positive and in control. Help the clients to prepare for the future.

— Helping others to protect themselves from HIV through education and condom distribution can make people with HIV feel valued and positive. However, it is important not to pressure them to take this role.

— Help people not to feel guilty about their HIV status.

Counselling HIV Negative Clients

- — Help clients to understand that a negative result only means that the test has not detected any antibodies. Help them to consider the possibility that they could be infected and not yet showing antibodies to HIV.
- — Ask clients whether they have engaged in any risky sexual activity over the past three months. If they have, suggest that they avoid any risky sex from now on and have another test in three months time or longer. They should act as if they are HIV positive until they get the results of repeat test.
- — Give all clients the opportunity to repeat the test to be sure of the result if they wish.

Psychological support: Clients may respond in a range of ways to a negative test result. Do not assume that clients will react with relief and happiness to a negative test result.

The risk reduction plan: If the client made a risk reduction plan at pre-test counselling, talk it over and ask: "How do you feel about your risk reduction plan now? Do you need to revise it?" If clients tell that they will stay safe by not having sex anymore, acknowledge their intention, but help them to have sufficient skills and a plan to protect themselves if they do have sex. For clients who came for a test without their sexual partners, discuss whether they intend to tell their partner that they were tested and how they will discuss safer sex or testing with their partner if necessary.

When a woman is HIV negative and the sero-status of her partner is unknown, the woman needs support to stay negative. If she can tell her partner and use this as an opportunity to encourage him to have a test also, this can be a big motivation for them both to practice safer sex from now on. The same thing applies if the man is negative.

Counselling when the Test Result is Not Clear

Sometimes the results of the test do not tell whether the test is positive or negative. This is frustrating for the client. This occurs rarely and may be because the person is in the pre-sero conversion phase. In this case, they should have a repeat test.

— Ask the client when they were last at risk of HIV infection. Ask them to come for a repeat test three months or longer after this date.

— Explain that the client needs to take the same precautions for reducing risk as a person testing HIV positive until the time of the repeat test.

Counselling Sexually-abused Clients

Both women and men can suffer from abuse related to sex, but generally men abuse women. For this reason, let us refer to the abused person as 'she' and the abuser as 'he', whilst recognising that males may also be abused by other men or women.

There may be several type of abuses in a relationship. They are:

— *Physical abuse* involves physical assault. It includes hitting, punching, kicking, pulling hair and throwing things at someone. It can result in permanent injury, disability and death. In most cases men use it to frighten women so that they can control them.

— *Sexual abuse* is where a person forces another to have sexual intercourse or other activities against their will; inflicts pain during sex or does not allow the partner to use contraception or protection against STI/HIV. This can result in emotional trauma, illness and death.

— *Sexual harassment* includes making unwanted sexual comments, touches or propositions.

— *Psychological abuse* includes threats of suicide, violence or taking the children away, destruction of property or precious things or making a person perform degrading or dangerous acts.
— *Economic abuse* includes keeping partners short of money for basic needs, stopping her getting a job or forcing her to do sex work; controlling the money and spending it on his own desires; destruction of property and undermining partner's attempts to improve education.
— Economic exploitation includes manipulating someone to have sex they don't want with the offer of material rewards, jobs or basic needs.

Any of these forms of abuse can take place at home, in the workplace, in school, in public places or in religious institutions.

Sexual cultures and gender norms vary across ethnic groups and abuse, violence and coercion are viewed in different ways. In some cultures, married women are obliged to have sex with their husbands, whether they like it or not and rape in marriage does not exist in law; and men have a right to beat their wives if they step out of line. However, cultures are changing continuously and most countries have signed up to human rights agreements that everyone has a right to choice in sexual activity and to be protected from violence. Counsellors have a role in changing culture and promoting human rights and laws through counselling and linking up with health promotion activities and activist groups.

In 95 per cent of cases, the abuser is known to the abused and women are most likely to be abused at home. Women do not like to be forced to have sex they do not want. If a woman is crying, looking terrified or unhappy, she is not enjoying sex. Provocative clothes do not cause rape. Babies and elderly women are raped, most women who are raped are wearing everyday clothes that do not provoke. Getting aroused without having sex does not harm men. Men can switch off arousal by thinking about or doing something else. They may get pain in their testicles but this goes away without harming them.

Nobody deserves to be physically hurt, however they behave. There is no excuse for violence. Abuse is not a sign of love. It hurts and damages the person being abused and kills love. Sexual abuse happens between people of all races, cultures, sexual orientation, economic status, religion, age and ability. It is difficult for women to leave abusive relationships for many reasons. These include economic dependency, fear, nowhere else to go, fear of losing the children and breaking up the family and unwillingness to admit that the marriage is not working and lose the status of a wife.

Many people do not know these facts and use misconceptions about abuse as an excuse for it. This makes it hard for survivors to get the support and help they need. They also make women blame themselves and not demand their rights. The counsellor can discuss these issues with survivors, families and communities and help to challenge their own misconceptions about themselves and their situation.

Links between abuse and STI/HIV, unwanted pregnancy and pregnancy mishaps include:

— Forced vaginal or anal sex easily tears the lining of the vagina or anus and this makes it easier for HIV or STI to be transmitted into the body.

— Women fear rejection and violence if they discuss ways to protect themselves from STI including HIV and partners refuse to use condoms consistently or at all.

— Men who know that they have an STI or HIV do not tell their wives or girlfriends.

— Women are blamed for bringing HIV and/or STI into a relationship. If they disclose their HIV status, they risk scorn, rejection and violence.

— Many married women are forced to have sex with their husbands in spite of fears about pregnancy or HIV.

— Many married women are infected with HIV by their husbands.

— For many girls, first sex is forced. HIV incidence is six times higher in girls than boys.

— Women fear discussing, or are unable to use, contraception or natural family planning methods to plan their pregnancies; they have unplanned pregnancies leading to unsafe abortions or higher risk in childbirth. Refusal to have sex because of a wish to avoid pregnancy is a common cause of violence.

— Abused women are more likely to have miscarriages and premature births.

— Women who are abused suffer from gynaecological symptoms such as chronic pelvic pain more frequently.

Helping clients to talk about abuse

— *Be aware* that any one of the clients may be in an abusive relationship or have been abused and this will affect how you can help them. Spousal consent policies or discussions about condoms may put abused women at risk of violence. A pregnant 14-year-old girl or a woman with chronic pelvic pain may have been raped.

— *Look out for symptoms of abuse and screen* clients for physical or sexual abuse, provide initial counselling and refer them to available services.

— Open up the conversation about the client's sexual relationship

Use questions like:

— What might make it difficult for you to protect yourself from unwanted pregnancy and infection?

— How might your partner respond if you talk to him about contraception or safe sex?

— Does your partner want sex more often than you want it? Has he ever pressured or forced you to have sex when you didn't want it?

— What happens if you say that you do not want to have sex?

— Has your partner or anyone else tried to physically harm you in any way?

— Did you have any upsetting experiences in childhood or adolescence?

With this understanding, the counsellor can help the client in the most appropriate way. For example, explore together ways to minimise the risk of abuse when using contraception or talking about safer sex practices or disclosing an STI or HIV result. Reaffirm confidentiality by making sure that the client knows that what she or he says will not be repeated elsewhere. This is crucial because it can prevent further harm to the client. The counsellor need to get permission from the client before he/she refer her or him to another service, for example, a doctor or the police.

Ways to Empower the Client

Even if the counsellor cannot refer an abused client or offer much practical help, he/she can empower the client by:

— *Believing her story*: Listen actively, ask questions, empathise and avoid making judgements or giving advice.

— *Building on her strengths:* Complement her on what she has achieved so far, her coping strategies and survival skills. For example, in coming to see you. Help her to build on these strengths.

— *Validating her feelings:* Abused women often have mixed feelings about the abuser, for example, love, anger, hope, fear, sadness and guilt. Give the woman time and support to let out all her feelings. Let her know that they are normal and reasonable.

— *Avoid blaming her for the situation:* reinforce that the abuse is not her fault – it is the responsibility and problem of the perpetrator. Resist the temptation to criticise his personality, talk instead about his behaviour.

— *Take her fears seriously:* Listen and empathise with the client's fears and worries. Take them seriously, do not judge how serious a problem is. Discuss options to overcome these fears and worries.

— *Offer help:* Offer specific and appropriate forms of help and information. Do not make false promises and end up not being able to meet her needs.

Giving practical help: Network and refer clients to appropriate local services and groups. Link up with local services and women's groups. Provide information about these services in your clinic or talk to women in the community about them. Invite experienced people to train your counsellors and staff on helping abused women.

Pregnancy

— Help the client to talk with her partner about contraception if she wishes. Offer couple counselling or counselling for her partner. Provide print materials if appropriate.

— Help the client to use a contraceptive without her partners' knowledge if she feels that this is the only solution. Discuss potential difficulties, for example, changes in menstruation.

— Provide emergency contraception if the client has had unprotected forced sex within the past 72 hours.

— Offer a pregnancy test and discuss termination if it is legal and the client is interested.

STI and HIV

— Explore ways to talk with the partner about safer sex and rehearse them if appropriate. Consider asking other people to help, for example, a relative or friend of the partner.

— Consider the use of female condoms or microbicides, if available.

— Discuss having tests for STI and/or taking antibiotics.
— Discuss the HIV test and the use of prophylactic anti-retrovirals drugs if available.

The abusive relationship

— Discuss which trusted people might support the client to cope with the situation and make a plan for disclosure if appropriate.
— Discuss going to a lawyer and/or the police to take legal action.
— Discuss options to prevent or end an abusive situation and help the client to decide on the best course of action.

Options might be:

— To leave the partner and situation and live with a supportive person or in a refuge;
— To obtain more support from others in changing the partner's behaviour, for example, community leaders, mediators, friends or relatives.
— Counselling the perpetrator individually or as a couple.
— Small group counselling or skills building activities to explore relationships, communication and ways of improving them.
— Recognising and avoiding or addressing triggers which result in abuse, for example, alcohol.
— Supporting the client to ask the law to intervene.
— Building the client's support network to put pressure on the abuser to change and to respond in abusive episodes.
— Link up with or initiate community work aimed at changing sexual and gender norms.
— Counsel the members of the abused person's family also.
— Consider the pros and cons of each option. This will help the client to make an informed decision. Do not expect a quick solution to the problem of abuse, even if frustrated. It often takes time for a woman to work through her

feelings and options. Even then, she may decide that the best option is to stay in the abusive relationship and do nothing.

— Explore the effects of all the partner's forms of controlling behaviour on the client. Do not hold the client responsible for the abuse in any way or encourage her to change as a way of getting the abuser to change.
— Be prepared to challenge your own attitudes and ideas about abused clients.
— Support the client to choose what action she wants to take. Agree on a follow-up and feedback strategy before she leaves.

Counselling to Prevent Parent-to-Child Transmission of HIV/AIDS

HIV can be transmitted from an infected mother to her child during pregnancy, delivery and breast-feeding. Transmission ranges from 15-25 per cent in rich countries to 25-45 per cent in resource poor countries. The extra risk of HIV infection when an infant is breast-fed is around 15 per cent. There are a number of interventions that can reduce the risk of transmission to as low as 10 per cent. The health, well-being and sexuality of mothers as women is important, so counsel them on all the issues of safer sex when they attend services, not just pregnancy and preventing transmission to the child.

The prevention of HIV transmission to Pregnant Women, Mothers and their Children (PMTCT) includes:

— The prevention of HIV infection in women, mothers and mothers-to-be;
— The prevention of unwanted pregnancies;
— The prevention of HIV transmission from the infected mother to the infant.

The prevention of HIV in men and women of child-bearing age is a very important strategy for individuals, couples and communities as well as counsellors. Safe sexual behaviour and fast treatment of STI greatly reduces risk of transmission to children. Men have a major responsibility to practice safe sex and inform their female partners if they are at risk of STI. Women need awareness of the benefits of condoms and the ability to negotiate safer sex. Family planning counsellors are key to the prevention of unwanted pregnancies. Making contraceptives, emergency contraception and safe abortion, accessible to all women, rich or poor, young or old, unmarried or single would reduce the rate of transmission to infants.

Prevention of transmission of HIV through pregnancy and breast-feeding involves:

- — STI screening and treatment.
- — Accessible, high quality Voluntary Counselling and Testing (VCT) for mothers and fathers.
- — Safe sex during pregnancy and breast-feeding.
- — Prophylactic treatment by anti-retroviral drugs.
- — Avoidance of invasive obstetrical procedures.
- — Alternatives to early mixed feeding and prolonged breast-feeding.
- — Safe sex after delivery to prevent unwanted pregnancies.

These options require high quality ante-natal care (ANC) and VCT, care during delivery, post-natal care for mother and child and counselling on infant feeding. If VCT is promoted, it is an ethical imperative to ensure that women who are HIV positive have access to long-term care and support. The advantages of VCT before, during and after delivery depend on the availability of treatment, the possibility of safer sex and support.

Counselling before conception

Some women and men may wish to know their HIV-status before considering conception. Some women and men who know that they are HIV positive may wish to discuss issues around having a child before they consider pregnancy. Some women and men who have lost their babies due to HIV may wish to have another child.

Counselling before conception could include:

— Voluntary testing for one or both partners
— Counselling on the positive and negative points in conceiving at this time
— Counselling about reasons for wanting to conceive a baby when the woman and/or her partner is HIV positive.
— Minimising the risk of HIV transmission in becoming pregnant.
— Risks of mother to child transmission and options to prevent PMTCT.
— Increased risk of PMTCT if HIV contracted during pregnancy and breast-feeding.
— Long-term outcome for mother and baby, including ill-health, stigma and loss of parents.
— STI diagnosis and treatment.
— STI and HIV prevention in pregnancy, safer sex for both partners.
— Need to attend early for antenatal care to benefit fully.

Counselling pregnant women and their partners

If a mother is infected with HIV during pregnancy or breast-feeding, the risk of transmission to the infant is high because the amount of virus in the blood and milk is high. STI in pregnancy also increase the risk of PMTCT. Counsel women, and if possible, their partners during pregnancy and lactation, so that they understand the importance of avoiding HIV infection and STI and put risk reduction plans in place.

Women at antenatal clinics have the same rights to informed consent and need the same pre-test counselling as clients in any other setting. Help them to think through the advantages and disadvantages of testing in relation to the baby as well as their own lives. Do not promote testing and be honest about the support that can offer if the result is positive.

Advantages

- — Know, understand and are helped to cope with HIV status.
- — Empowered to make good choices about having the baby or termination.
- — Access to appropriate health care for mother and child.
- — Access to information about negotiating for safer sex.
- — Support with prevention of HIV transmission (for those testing negative and positive).
- — To help partner share her HIV status.
- — Gain access to ongoing support (social and emotional) through shared confidentiality.

Disadvantages

- — Emotional distress.
- — Stigma.
- — Abuse or abandonment by partner.
- — Breached confidentiality.
- — Frustration if no treatment or support is available.

Counselling for HIV positive woman

Telling partners about the test result: It is often particularly difficult for a woman tested at the antenatal clinic to inform her partner she is positive soon after getting the result. Her partner and family may blame her for bringing the infection into the family although the status of her partner is unknown and he may have infected her. This can have a long-lasting negative impact on her psychosocial and economic well-being and family life. Testing at antenatal clinics can make people see HIV and AIDS as a woman's disease. In some settings, counselling and testing partners together is very helpful. In others, couples do not wish to be tested together. It is important to provide VCT in settings where men feel comfortable.

Counselling on continuation of pregnancy: Women who test HIV positive in early pregnancy in countries where abortion is safe and legal, may wish to discuss whether to continue the pregnancy or have a termination.

Methods to prevent mother to child transmission: Talk to clients about the available treatment and care options for prevention of Mother to Child Transmission so that they can make informed decisions relating to their pregnancy. If the counsellor can offer or refer for ARV treatments, informed consent, detailed explanations, monitoring and follow-up are particularly important, as the procedure is complex. It may involve a number of different services, including family planning and infant feeding support. It is essential that the client takes the drugs correctly. The counsellor can help the client to do this if he understands the regime, the risks and benefits.

Mothers who have ARV treatment should not breast-feed their infants because the drug goes into her breast milk and may harm the baby. The feasibility and safety of alternative infant feeding in the mother's particular circumstances may determine whether she decides to have ARV treatment. The number of infants of mothers receiving short course ARV treatment who contract HIV is greatly reduced to around 10 per cent. These infected infants need continuing medical care and they, their mothers and families need social and emotional support.

Women with HIV often worry about what is going to happen to their children if they become sick or die. These worries are not specific to women testing during the antenatal period but health workers must be open to discussing them at this time. Women may need help with planning for the future and advice to help them prevent "property grabbing". They may be anxious or depressed about what the future holds, especially if they have seen friends or relatives dying from AIDS. Health workers should keep up to date about the existing and potential availability of ARV drugs to treat the mother in the longer term. They should be able to refer for spiritual and legal support if available.

REFERENCES

Academy for Educational Development, *Fundamentals of HIV Prevention Counselling: Participants Manual*, 1998.

EngenderHealth, *STI/HIV Prevention – Quick Reference Cards for Health Care Providers – What Every Client Should Know*, New York,2001.

Gordon, G. and Gordon, P., *Counselling and Sexuality: A Video Based Training Resource*, IPPF, London, 1992.

Ndondo, Noziqhu. T., "Preventing mother-to-child transmission of HIV. A training manual for healthcare providers", *Reproductive Health Alliance*, London, 2001.

Programme guidance on Counselling for STI/HIV prevention in sexual and reprodu ctive health settings, International Planned Parenthood Federation (IPPF), 2002.

South African AIDS Training (SAT) Programme, *Basic counselling guidelines in HIV and AIDS*, July, 2001.

____________ *Counselling Guidelines on Disclosure of HIV Status*, 2001.

____________ *Counselling Guidelines on Domestic Violence*, April, 2001.

____________ *Counselling Guidelines on Child Sexual Abuse*, 2001.

The Bangkok Collaborative Perinatal HIV Transmission Study Group, *Counselling Pregnant Women and New Mothers about HIV*, Produced by the HIV/AIDS Collaboration, Thailand, 1999.

UNAIDS, *Counselling and voluntary HIV testing for pregnant women in high prevalence countries: Guidance for service providers*, May, 1999.

____________ , *Opening up the HIV epidemic: Guidance on encouraging beneficial disclosure, ethical partner counselling, and appropriate use of HIV case reporting*. Geneva: UNAIDS, 2001.

Welbourn, A., "Stepping Stones: A Training Package on HIV/AIDS, communication and relationship skills", *Strategies for Hope*, 1995.

5

Infant Feeding

Today, a large number of children are infected with the Human Immunodeficiency Virus (HIV). The overwhelming source of HIV infection in young children is mother-to-child transmission. The virus may be transmitted during pregnancy, labour and delivery, or by breast-feeding. HIV transmission may continue for as long as a child is breast-fed. Among women recently infected with HIV, the risk of transmission through breast-feeding is nearly twice as high as for women infected before or during pregnancy, because of high viral load shortly after initial infection.

The risks associated with not breast-feeding vary according to the environment, for example with the availability of suitable replacement feeds and safe water. It also varies with the individual circumstances of the mother and her family, including her education and economic status. Lack of breast-feeding compared to any breast-feeding has been expose children to increased risk of malnutrition and life-threatening infectious diseases other than HIV, especially in the first year of life, and exclusive breastfeeding appears to offer greater protection against disease than any breast-feeding.

In developing countries 54 per cent of all under-five deaths are associated with malnutrition. Not breast-feeding during the first two months of life is also associated, in poor countries, with a six-fold increase in mortality due to infectious diseases. This increased risk drops to two-and-a-half-fold at six months, and continues to decrease with time. Mothers who do not breast-feed, or who stop breast-feeding early, are more likely to become pregnant again rapidly, and this has implications for their health and that of their infants.

WHO reviewed the evidence and concluded that "the new results do not warrant any change in current policies on breast-feeding, nor on infant feeding by HIV-infected women." However, they "emphasise the need for proper support to mothers who are infected with HIV and provide a further reason for women to know their HIV infection status".

According to UN, infants should be exclusively breast-fed for the first six months of life to achieve optimal growth, development and health. Thereafter, infants should receive nutritionally adequate and safe complementary foods while breast-feeding continues up to 24 months or beyond. However, given the need to reduce the risk of HIV transmission to infants while minimising the risk of other causes of morbidity and mortality, the guidelines also state that "when replacement feeding is acceptable, feasible, affordable, sustainable and safe, avoidance of all breast-feeding by HIV-infected mothers is recommended".

Otherwise, exclusive breast-feeding is recommended during the first months of life and should then be discontinued as soon as it is feasible. To help HIV-positive mothers make the best choice, they should receive counselling that includes information about both the risks and benefits of various infant feeding options based on local assessments, and guidance in selecting the most suitable option for their situation. They should also have access to follow-up care and support, including family planning and nutritional support. For an individual mother, balancing risks and benefits is a complex, but necessary, task.

HIV-positive mothers being provided with counselling on infant feeding options, there should be an effort to ensure positive perceptions of and attitudes towards breast-feeding within the general population. In addition, the unnecessary use of breast-milk substitutes by mothers who do not know their

HIV sero-status or who are HIV-negative should be avoided. All such mothers should be encouraged and supported to breast-feed exclusively for six months, and continue breast-feeding with complementary feeding until 24 months as this practice is best for their overall health and that of their children. Through this combined approach, it should be possible to achieve the ultimate goal of increasing overall child survival, while reducing HIV infection in infants and young children.

During the United Nations General Assembly Special Session (UNGASS) for Children, governments pledged to reduce infant and under-five mortality by at least one-third during the decade 2001-2010, and by two-thirds by 2015. Governments also declared they would take action consistent with the June 2001 UNGASS on HIV/AIDS, to reduce the proportion of the infant population infected with HIV by 20 per cent by 2005, and by 50 per cent by 2010. To achieve these goals, the UN strategic approach for preventing the transmission of HIV to women and their children includes four areas:

i) prevention of HIV infection in general, especially in young women, and in pregnant women;
ii) prevention of unintended pregnancies among HIV-infected women;
iii) prevention of HIV transmission from HIV-infected mothers to their infants; and provision of care, treatment and support to HIV-infected women, their infants and family.

The *Global Strategy for Infant and Young Child Feeding* was adopted by the World Health Assembly in May 2002 and by the UNICEF Board in September 2002. The operational objectives of this strategy include: ensuring that exclusive breast-feeding is protected, promoted and supported for six months, with continued breast-feeding up to two years and beyond; promoting timely, adequate, safe and appropriate complementary feeding; and providing guidance on feeding infants and young children in exceptionally difficult circumstances, e.g., for infants of HIV-infected women, in emergency situations and for low birth-weight babies. The current framework has been developed in accordance with the goals and strategies of this integrated policy context.

HIV and infant feeding is a complex issue, and there are still significant knowledge gaps, including whether anti-retroviral prophylaxis for an infant during breast-feeding, or anti-retroviral treatment for a breast-feeding mother, are safe and effective in reducing HIV transmission. Identification and implementation of good practices requires a comprehensive approach in the context of a broad strategy, such as that described above. In addition it will require an enabling environment where appropriate infant and young child feeding is the norm and efforts to address broader issues of food security for HIV-affected families are in place.

COUNSELLING FOR SAFER INFANT FEEDING

When an HIV-positive woman breast-feeds her infant, a further 5-20 per cent risk of transmission is added. Among 672 infants (HIV-negative at birth) born to HIV-positive mothers in Malawi, 47 (7 per cent) sero-converted while breast-feeding. The cumulative infection rate while breast-feeding at 5, 11, 17, and 23 months was 3.5 per cent, 7.0 per cent, 8.9 per cent, and 10.3 per cent, respectively. Monthly incidence was 0.7 per cent from 1-5 months, 0.6 per cent from 6-11 months, and 0.3 per cent from 12-17 months.

Thus, the risk for breast milk transmission is highest in the early months of life the time when infants are most susceptible to morbidity from enteric infections from contaminated feeds. This has created a public health dilemma in resource-constrained settings, where breast-feeding is the primary guarantee for child health, development, and survival, particularly in the early months of life.

Replacement feeding means the process of feeding a child who is not receiving any breast milk with a diet that provides all the nutrients the child needs. During the first six months this should be with a suitable BMS-commercial formula, or home-prepared formula with micronutrient supplements.

After six months, preferably feed a suitable BMS, and complementary foods made from appropriately prepared and nutrient-enriched family foods, given four times a day. If suitable BMSs are not available, feed appropriately prepared family foods that are further enriched, given four times a day. Breast-feeding and feeding BMSs at the same time (mixed feeding) is the most dangerous option for the baby. This practice exposes the baby to all the disadvantages of replacement feeding as well as increased risk of HIV infection from breast milk.

Guidance on Optimal Breast-feeding

In most developing countries breast-feeding is nearly universal and is the normative infant feeding method.

The major benefits of breast-feeding are given below.

i) reduces infant morbidity and mortality associated with infectious diseases, particularly diarrhoea and respiratory infections. This is especially important for younger infants of women who are more disadvantaged and have less education. These infants may experience up to five to six times more illness and death from diarrhoea, respiratory infections, and other infectious disease in the absence of breast-feeding.

ii) provides perfect nutrition and is the natural food for newborns and young infants.

iii) bonds mother and child.

iv) inexpensive and readily available.

v) stimulates uterine contractions immediately postpartum, thus helping to stop postpartum bleeding and stimulates uterine involution (shrinking to pre-pregnant size) in the first few weeks postpartum.

vi) benefits the mother by birth spacing, facilitating involution of the uterus after delivery, hence reducing the risk of postpartum haemorrhage, and protecting against certain cancers.

Some disadvantages of breast-feeding are:

i) Risk of postnatal transmission of HIV.
ii) Only the mother can feed the baby (unless a suitable wet nurse is available).
iii) May increase maternal mortality rate in HIV-infected mothers

Factors that increase HIV transmission from mother-to-child are:

i) Sero-conversion (acquiring initial infection) during lactation
ii) Bleeding or cracked nipples
iii) Subclinical and clinical mastitis
iv) Breast abscesses
v) Mixed feeding
vi) Open sores in infant's mouth

This highlights the need for proper instruction of mothers in good breast-feeding techniques, the practice of exclusive breast-feeding, prompt treatment for breast conditions, and avoidance of HIV infection for those who are not infected, or whose status is unknown. This enables HIV-infected mothers who choose to breast-feed, and those whose status is unknown, to breast-feed optimally with less risk of HIV transmission through breast milk.

Some guidance on optimal breast-feeding for mothers are given below:

i) *If the baby is not positioned correctly*

— Baby's tummy is not flat against mother's

Show the mother correct positioning

— Baby is facing mother and is close to her.

— Baby's tummy is flat against mother's tummy.

ii) *If the not properly attached to the breast*

— Baby looks like is sucking a straw.

— Baby's mouth does not cover areola.

Show the mother correct attachment

— Baby's chin is touching the breast.

— Baby's mouth covers all the areola (dark skin around the nipple).

— Baby's lower lip is curled outward.

An HIV-positive mother who chooses to breast-feed should be supported to maintain exclusive breast-feeding and to wean her infant early (no later than six months). As much as possible, a period of mixed feeding should be avoided or kept to the absolute minimum through "rapid weaning."

Weaning and Reducing Breast Engorgement

"Abrupt weaning" can cause the baby to be fussy and to feed poorly, and cause the mother to have painful breast engorgement. Breast engorgement can lead to plugged milk ducts, mastitis, and breast abscesses, if not treated correctly. One must balance the danger of increased HIV transmission from brief mixed feeding against the risks of poor feeding and breast engorgement from abrupt weaning. Therefore, it may be most acceptable to wean over the course of about two weeks (rapid weaning). Although abrupt weaning is optimal practice, it is advisable to work with each mother to achieve weaning safely over as short a time as possible.

Rapid Weaning

i) Express breast milk and give to baby using a cup, especially during the day.

ii) At first, continue to breast-feed during the night, to assure adequate rest for mother and baby.

iii) Increase the number of expressed breast milk feeds from the cup, while decreasing the number of feeds directly from the breast gradually over a two-week period.

iv) Learn how to prepare animal milk or commercial infant formula

v) Stop breast-feeding as soon as possible when the baby is used to feeding from the cup.

vi) Introduce complementary foods when baby is six months old.

Reducing Breast Engorgement in Abrupt or Rapid Weaning

i) *Do*: Wear a bra or breast binder that presses firmly against the nipples. It may help to put gauze or clean cloth over the nipples, under the bra cup or breast binder, to absorb dripping milk and add pressure on the nipples. If engorgement is severe or painful, briefly remove or loosen bra or binder and allow milk to drip, unstimulated. In extreme cases, it may be necessary to express a small amount of milk. Use mild analgesics, such as paracetamol, aspirin, or ibuprofen as needed for pain.

ii) Taking combination estrogen/progesterone birth control pills may decrease milk production in mothers who are trying to wean. However, starting combination birth control pills prior to two-three weeks postpartum is not recommended, because the estrogen may slightly increase the mother's hypercoagulable state.

iii) Some have suggested applying washed cabbage leaves over the breasts, under the bra or binder, changing them twice a day, and leaving the nipple free. There is insufficient evidence for or against the effectiveness of this method.

iv) *Do not*: Use any type of nipple stimulation (squeezing, sucking, massaging), as this will promote lactation.

v) *Do not*: Reduce fluid intake or take diuretics, as this is dangerous to the mother, especially in the immediate postpartum period or if she has been working or engaging in vigorous physical activity.

Women Choosing Not to Breast-feed-Replacement Feeding

i) Because of the complexity of the issues involved, counsel all HIV-infected mothers about the risks and benefits of various infant feeding options and provide specific guidance in selecting the most suitable option.

ii) When replacement feeding is acceptable, feasible, affordable, sustainable, and safe, WHO recommends that all HIV infected mothers not breast-feed. Otherwise, exclusive breast-feeding is recommended during the first six months of life.

iii) To minimise the risk of HIV transmission, breast-feeding should be discontinued as soon as feasible, taking into account local circumstances, the individual woman's situation, and the risks of replacement feeding (including infections other than HIV and malnutrition)

Infant Feeding Options

HIV can be transmitted from mother to child through breast-feeding. The extra risk of HIV infection when an infant is breast-fed is around 15 per cent. HIV transmission during breast-feeding is increased by the factors in the following table which also shows ways to reduce risk.

Factors increasing risk

— Recent infection with HIV during pregnancy or while breast-feeding

— The mother has AIDS
— Infection with STIs
— Vitamin A deficiency
— Cracked or bleeding nipples or breast abscess
— Other foods and drinks given with breast-milk
— Longer duration of breast-feeding

Way to reduce risk

— Counsel mother or couple about safer sex during pregnancy and breast-feeding.
— If the mother develops AIDS during pregnancy or breast-feeding, try to find a replacement food
— Screen and treat mothers for STI. Counsel on safer sex.
— Provide Vitamin A supplements or teach mother how to obtain from local foods.
— Counsel on management of breast-feeding and treat.
— Give only breast-milk with no other food and drink, including water, for the first six months. Stop breast-feeding completely at six months and switch to other foods/substitutes.

Infant feeding from birth to six months: Breast milk is normally the best food for an infant. If the mother is HIV positive, replacement feeding may be best to reduce the risk of HIV transmission. However, for each mother, the health risks of replacement feeding should be less than the risk of HIV infection. ARV drug treatment, if the mother is considering ARV to prevent Mother to Child Transmission, explain that if she chooses to have ARV treatment, she should not breast-feed her infant because the drug goes into her breast milk and may harm the baby. The feasibility and safety of alternative infant feeding in her particular circumstances may determine whether she decides to have ARV treatment

The risks of replacement include:

— Malnutrition
— Infection
— High cost
— Loss of child spacing
— Loss of mother-child bonding
— Stigmatisation of mother.

Some ways to reduce the risks are given below:

— Ensure that family have enough breast-milk substitute for six months.
— Teach hygiene rules that will work in living conditions of mother.
— Subsidise or provide free.
— Counsel the couple on contraception.
— Counsel the parents/family on ways to give child attention.
— Counsel partner and family to support mother.
— Work to change community attitudes.

From birth to six months, milk in some form is essential for an infant. If not breast-fed, an infant needs about 150 ml of milk per KG of body weight a day.

Before the counsellor start his job on infant feeding, he can find out the options available in the locality he work and how safe they are likely to be, the social and economic conditions and local infant feeding practices.

Counselling both parents and/or other members of the family may make it easier for the mother to choose the best way to feed her infant without fear of stigma, if they can accept her HIV status.

Breast-milk substitutes: These might be commercial infant formula, home prepared modified animal milk, dried milk powder or evaporated milk or unmodified cow's milk. Non-commercial breast-milk substitutes should only be considered when families do not have access to commercial substitutes. If they are not using commercial formula, they will need to learn how to modify the milk and to give micronutrient supplements.

Table 1

Guidance on breast milk substitutes and modified breast-feeding

Breast milk substitutes	
Options	*Requirements*
Commercial baby formula	Financial means for 20 kg of powdered milk or 44 tins of 450g or 40 tins of 500 g: (80,000 CFAs or US$133) for 6 months. Potable water and adequate level of education.
Animal milk	Whole animal milk not recommended before age 12 months. Modified animal milk not ideal, but sometimes is the only option
Modified Breast-feeding	
Early discontinuation of breast- -feeding (especially important in mothers with AIDS or TB)	Optimal date of cessation determined. Every mother wanting to stop must have substitute available.
Heating of breast milk to 62.5°C for 30 minutes	Pasteurised milk of higher nutritive value than others. Disadvantage: Destroys immune globulins that would protect the baby against infection. Highly motivated mother required.
Feeding by a wet nurse	HIV-negative wet nurse fully informed of baby's HIV status and of possible risk of infection in case of nipple cracks, if baby is HIV-positive.

Skimmed and sweetened condensed milk, yoghurt, fruit juices, sugar water and dilute cereal gruels are not suitable for feeding infants under six months of age.

Families with enough income or access to free commercial breast-milk substitutes to provide sufficient milk for six months, with a good water supply, sanitation system, and supportive family and community members are most likely to be able to stop breast-feeding and give substitutes safely.

Modified breast-feeding: If the mother chooses to breast-feed, it is best to give breast-milk only with no other liquids, including water, or foods because this prevents infection of both HIV and other diseases. If breast milk and substitutes are given, the baby is more at risk from both HIV and other infections. It has been found that exclusive breast-feeding for six months and then completely stopping reduces Mother to Child Transmission. Mothers with HIV infection could consider this as an option if they:

— Find it difficult for social reasons to avoid breast-feeding altogether.

— Develop symptoms of AIDS during the breast-feeding period.

— Can only provide safe and adequate replacement feeds after their baby is six months old.

— Heating breastmilk kills HIV. Expressing and heat-treating breast milk is time consuming and may not be a practical option for mothers at home.

— Breast milk banks are not an option for meeting infant needs over a long period. They need to have high standards of screening and pasteurising for the milk to be safe.

— In wet-nursing, there is a risk of HIV infection from wet-nurse to infant and from infant to wet-nurse, if either is infected with HIV. Clients should only consider it if the wet nurse has an HIV test and is uninfected; she is informed of the risks; she practises safer sex; she can breast feed the infant frequently enough and she has access to support to avoid cracked nipples.

Feeding children aged six months to two years: Breastmilk continues to be an important source of nutrients from six months to two years. If the mother stops breast-feeding at six months to reduce the risk of HIV infection, family foods need to be enriched with protein, energy and micro-nutrients and given five times a day.

Caveats on Replacement Feeding

i) Powdered, commercially made infant formula
   a) Lacks protective maternal immunoglobulins.
ii) Heat-treated (pasteurised) expressed breast milk from the mother
   a) May lose some immunoglobulins during pasteurisation process.
   b) Experience from South Africa and Zimbabwe shows that heating breast milk is technically very demanding and difficult, and would take an exceptional mother to adhere to this modification of breast-feeding.
iii) Breast milk from an uninfected wet nurse
   a) Wet nurses who are willing to be tested for HIV may be difficult to find.
iv) Animal milk
   a) Whole, unmodified cow milk is not recommended before age 12 months, because of its high solute load, low iron content, and risk of causing intestinal bleeding, leading to anaemia.
   b) Modified animal milk, diluted with water and with added sugar, lacks iron, zinc, and other essential micronutrients. More research is needed to determine the effect on growth and nutritional adequacy, especially before age six months.

c) Consider animal milk pre-diluted by a vendor to be unsafe, unless the mother is sure the vendor follows the instructions below.

Counselling Mothers on Replacement Feeding

i) *Time*: Begin counselling HIV-positive mothers on infant feeding options either at the time the counsellor inform them of a positive test result or soon thereafter, and continue counselling on each subsequent antenatal visit. If a mother who plans not to breast-feed has just delivered, counsel her and, if possible, other family members before she leaves the hospital. If she is already breast-feeding, determine when she plans to stop. Ask if this is a good time to discuss replacement feeding.

ii) *Place*: (ideally, counselling should occur in a setting where the counsellor can demonstrate food preparation techniques):

   a) In private counselling room in clinic

   b) During home visit

   c) During support group meetings

iii) Feasibility:

   a) Will she leave her baby in care of someone else while she goes to work?

   b) Is there a responsible baby carer who will be able to safely prepare replacement feeds?

   c) Can she afford replacement feeds?

   d) Are adequate firewood, water sources, and dishes available to prepare boiled water and clean containers?

iv). Type of replacement feed available in her local community:

   a) Commercial infant formula.

   b) Animal milk (use whole milk, not milk diluted by vendor).

c) Liquid porridge. Most such preparations are nutritionally inadequate as a sole food source.

v) *Traditional practices*: It is critical to make counselling as culturally appropriate as possible, to take advantage of helpful practices, and to find culturally sensitive ways of discouraging harmful practices:

a) Is mixed feeding the norm, especially when the mother returns to work on their farms?

b) Is liquid porridge commonly given to infants? Animal milk?

c) Are foods softened by premastication or other techniques to add nutrients to infant feeds? Are infants given liquid from boiled foods, such as stews?

d) Is wet-nursing practised? Are there certain women designated to be wet nurses?

e) If there a customary carer (e.g., mother-in-law), and has the mother disclosed her HIV status?

Preparing Animal Milk

Although animal milk is not ideal, it is the only option for many mothers. When possible, additional sources of vitamins and minerals should be added.

i) Have ready the following materials:

a) Fresh, clean animal milk

b) Boiled, clean water (potable water)

c) 2-litre jar with a tight cover

d) 2 cups without covers

e) 1 larger, clear, marked container to measure 100 mls

f) 1 teaspoon

g) Clean mat or other material on which to place the clean utensils

h) 2 teaspoonfuls of sugar for each feeding

ii) Have the mother prepare the milk as below. Explain, observe, correct errors, praise success.

a) If she uses undiluted, fresh cow, goat, or camel milk:
— Wash hands and utensils with soap and clean water
— Measure 100 ml of milk
— Put the milk into a clean jug
— Add 50 ml of clean, boiled water that has cooled
— Add 2 teaspoonfuls of sugar
— Mix and boil the milk
— Let the milk cool
— Measure amount to feed baby

b) If she uses undiluted, fresh sheep or buffalo milk, modify the process:
— Measure 50 ml of milk
— Add 50 ml of potable cool water
— Add 1 teaspoon of sugar

Preparing Commercial Infant Formula

i) Follow instructions on formula package.
ii) Prepare clean boiled water and utensils.

Advantages of Replacement Feeding

i) May reduce maternal mortality.
ii) Eliminates the risk of HIV infection to the baby through breast milk.
iii) The infant can be fed by someone else.

Disadvantages of Replacement Feeding

i) Carries other health risks for the baby, especially if feeding involves the use of feeding bottles and unsafe water or if formula is mixed incorrectly due to inability to comprehend instructions.

ii) May lead to rationing because of the cost of formula, fuel, soap, thermos, cup, spoon, and other supplies.

iii) Illness and death from diarrhoea, respiratory problems, and other infectious diseases is up to five or six times higher in the first two months of an infant's life when not breast-fed

iv) Discrimination toward the mother by family and community, and possible inadvertent disclosure of HIV status.

Making Replacement Feeding Easier and Safer

i) For each mother giving breast milk substitutes, explain how to use a cup to feed her baby. Mention that using a spoon to feed the baby is too slow and may discourage the mother and baby.

ii) Tell the mother to feed the baby using an open cup following the steps below:

Step 1: Hold the baby upright or almost upright on your lap.

Step 2: Hold the cup of milk to the baby's lips.

Step 3: Rest the cup lightly on the baby's bottom lip.

Step 4: Tilt the cup so that the milk just reaches the baby's lips.

Step 5: Hold the cup to the baby's lips and let the baby take the milk at his or her own pace.

Do not pour the milk into the baby's mouth.

iii) Observe the mother and correct any errors.

iv) Talk to the mother about how to prepare the breast milk substitute of choice. The health worker should refer to the instructions for preparation provided for commercial formulae. If the mother feeds the infant animal milk, use pasteurised or heat-treated milk.

Table 2

HIV and Infant feeding counselling guidelines in resource-poor communities

Situation	*Health worker guidelines*
Mother's status is unknown	Promote availability and use of confidential testing. Promote breast-feeding as safer than artificial feeding. Teach mother how to avoid exposure to HIV.
HIV-negative mother	Promote breast-feeding as safest infant feeding method (exclusive breast-feeding for first 6 months, introduction of appropriate complementary foods at about 6 months, and continued breast-feeding up to 24 months and beyond). Teach mother how to avoid exposure to HIV.
HIV-positive mother who is considering her feeding options	Treat with ARV drugs if feasible. Counsel mother on the safety, availability, and affordability of feasible infant feeding options. Help mother choose and provide safest available infant feeding methods. Teach mother how to avoid sexual transmission of HIV.
HIV-positive mother who chooses to breast-feed	Promote safer breast-feeding (exclusive breast-feeding for 3 to 6 months, prevention and treatment of breast problems of mothers and thrush in infants, and shortened duration of breast-feeding when replacements are safe and feasible). Treat with ARV drugs if feasible.
HIV-positive mother who chooses to feed artificially	Help mother choose the safest alternative infant feeding strategy (methods, timing, etc.). Support her in her choice (provide education on hygienic preparation, health care, family planning services, etc.).

Infant Feeding Guidelines

A variety of tools have been developed to help a counsellor guide a mother in making an infant feeding choice. The following table summarises common health worker guidelines for mothers with different HIV statuses.

Often, a mother's infant feeding choice will change over time, as she resolves conflicts between what she would like to do and what her circumstances dictate. A counsellor's role is to provide information on all options, guide the mother in making her choice, and support her in her choice.

The infant feeding counselling should be done in PMTCT programs:

— During group health discussions. It should include addressing maternal nutrition issues and breast care to prepare mothers for exclusive breastfeeding.

— During post-test counselling positive women and refer to the Cato Manor tool for facilitating infant feeding choice. During early labour as appropriate for HIV-positive women. In particular it is important to affirm the mother's feeding method of choice, and specifically to make sure she has everything needed for replacement feeding, if she does not intend to breastfeed.

— After delivery to support the mother in initiating her feeding choice. Mothers who choose to breast-feed should put their infants to the breast within 30 minutes of delivery.

— At follow-up clinic visits and during home visits to sustain/adhere to the feeding method of choice.

— Ongoing to avoid mixed feeding, by supporting the process of rapid weaning for breast-feeding mothers, and to promote the safe introduction of other appropriate foods for all mothers. Encourage HIV-positive mothers whose infants test HIV-negative (6 weeks PCR) to wean their infants as soon as possible after three months, and no later than 6 months.

— Provide mothers with subsequent opportunities beyond the initial counselling to ask questions and to revisit their choice. Support them to follow through with their choices.

REFERENCES

De Cock K.M., Fowler M.G., Mercier E, *et al,* "Prevention of mother-to-child HIV transmission in resource-poor countries–Translating research into pol policy and practice", *JAMA,* 2000; 283: 1175-82.

Dunn D.T., Newell M.L., Ades A.E., *et al,* "Risk of human immunodeficiency virus type 1 transmission through breastfeeding", *Lancet,* 1992, 340:585-8.

Global Programme on AIDS, "Consensus statement from the WHO/ UNICEF consultation on HIV transmission and breastfeeding", *Weekly Epidemiological Record,* 1992, 67:177–179.

Leroy V., Newell M.L., Dabis F., *et al.,* "International multicentre pooled analysis of late postnatal mother-to-child transmission of HIV-1 infection", *Lancet,* 1998. 352:597-600.

Nduati R., Richardson B.A., John G., *et al,* "Effect of breastfeeding on mortality among HIV-1 infected women: a randomised trial", *Lancet,* 2001, 357:1651-5.

Pelletier, D.L., Frongillo Jr. E.A., Habicht J.P.," Epidemiologic evidence for a potentiating effect of malnutrition on child mortality", *Am J Public Health,* 1993, 83:1130-33.

VanDerslice J., Popkin B., Bris Briscoe J., "Drinking-water qual quality, sanitation, and breastfeed breastfeeding: Their interactive effects on infant health", *Bull WHO,* 1994; 72(4):589-601.

UNAIDS, UNICEF and WHO. *HIV and infant feeding. A policy statement developed collaboratively by UNAIDS, UNICEF and WHO*, Geneva, UNAIDS, 1997.

______________ , *Prevention of HIV transmission from mother to child: meeting on planning for programme implementation,* Geneva, 23–24 March 1998.

Walker N, Schwärtlander B., Bryce J., "Meeting international goals in child survival and HIV/ AIDS", *Lancet,* 2002, 360:284-9.

WHO, *New data on the prevention of mother-to-child transmission of HIV and the policy implications: conclusions and recommendations,* WHO technical consultation on the behalf of the UNFPA/UNICEF/WHO/UNAIDS Inter-Agency Task Team on Mother-to-Child Transmission of HIV, Geneva, 11-13 October 2000.WHO/RHR/01.28

______________ , *Improving access to quality care in family planning: medical eligibility criteria for contraceptive use,* 2nd ed. Geneva, World Health Organisation, 2001.

6

Survival Guidance for HIV Patients

Presently, worldwide, it is estimated that over 33 million people are infected with HIV, and over 16 million have died of AIDS-related illnesses. In many resource-poor countries and among marginalised groups of people in industrialised countries, the number of new HIV infections continues to rise. In some countries in Africa, AIDS-related morbidity and mortality are causing major reversals in development, childhood mortality, and survival and life expectancy.

Realisation of the enormous impact that HIV/AIDS is having on the well-being of individuals, families and communities, forced governments and communities to review the effectiveness of their HIV/AIDS programmes. In the context of such reviews, some governments have considered whether the principles of confidentiality and informed consent contribute to the spread of HIV. There is concern that these principles allow a person who is HIV positive to keep his status confidential, and refuse to share it with sexual or drug-injecting partners, family members or the community.

Governments and others have asked whether these principles hinder efforts to prevent the spread of HIV and deny protection to the sexual and drug-injecting partners of those infected. There is also concern that the principle of confidentiality contributes to the "invisible" status of the epidemic and to the general denial of HIV/AIDS within communities and nations. As a result, policymakers have begun to consider legislation and practice that would allow breaches in confidentiality, mandatory partner notification and named HIV case-reporting for public health reasons; and would permit the criminal prosecution of individuals who are considered to have spread the virus deliberately.

To address these concerns, and in response to a request for WHO assistance made by Ministers of Health in Africa, WHO (AFRO) and the UNAIDS Secretariat cosponsored a regional technical consultation on notification, confidentiality and HIV/AIDS in August 1999 in Windhoek, Namibia. A meeting statement was produced that aimed to assist Ministers of Health and other partners in southern Africa to develop policy and guidelines. Further, in October 1999, the UNAIDS Secretariat and WHO cohosted an international consultation in Geneva, Switzerland, on HIV reporting and disclosure. This consultation included epidemiologists, public health officials, national AIDS programme managers, people with HIV/AIDS, lawyers and human rights activists from more than 20 countries. The Windhoek and Geneva meetings confirmed that the principles of confidentiality and informed consent do not contribute to the spread of HIV/AIDS. Indeed, if employed in the appropriate context and in creative and culturally sensitive ways, confidentiality and informed consent can help to decrease the spread of HIV/AIDS. Rather, responsibility lies with the denial, stigma and discrimination which continue to surround HIV/AIDS, and which result in a high level of secrecy concerning the epidemic.

This denial, stigma and discrimination, and the resulting secrecy, must be overcome and the HIV/AIDS epidemic normalised into what it is — a viral infection, as well as a major human, health and development crisis. Relevance of ethical principles such as confidentiality and informed consent has been raised throughout the history of the response to the epidemic. That these come under examination again at this stage is a necessary and welcome development. In general, it highlights the need for greater efforts to 'open up' the HIV/AIDS epidemic. In particular, it highlights the need to identify more clearly the causes and consequences of the denial, stigma, discrimination and secrecy that surround HIV/AIDS and hinder effective responses.

The denial, stigma, discrimination and secrecy regarding HIV/AIDS continue to exist even though prevalence of HIV, and deaths from AIDS, are very high in many places. They stem from several causes.

At the individual level, people do not want to acknowledge that HIV/AIDS is within their communities, that it poses a real personal threat to them and to their families, that they themselves may already be infected and that they may be transmitting the virus to their sexual or drug-injecting partners. Furthermore, people do not want to get tested for HIV or to disclose their HIV status because they fear that they will be rejected by their partners, that they will face stigma and discrimination, and/or that they will be blamed for infecting others. Finally, most people in the developing world know they will not have access to drugs and treatment which would slow down the progression of the disease or alleviate its pain and suffering. Thus, denial, stigma, discrimination and lack of access to care stem from, and lead to, a sense of fear and hopelessness, and encourage secrecy about HIV/AIDS.

At the community level, many resource-poor communities are struggling with extremely difficult conditions in which to combat HIV/AIDS. They suffer from insufficient health care and education services, including insufficient voluntary testing and counselling; insufficient public education campaigns, particularly education targeted to young people, women and marginalised groups; insufficient access not only to anti-retroviral drugs but also to drugs to reduce the pain and suffering caused by AIDS-related illnesses; and insufficient community organisation and support, including lack of a social and legal infrastructure to protect people from HIV-related discrimination. These conditions are exacerbated among marginalised groups in communities. These obstacles seriously hamper government and community efforts to prevent the spread of HIV and to provide care and support for those affected by HIV/AIDS.

Governments and communities have felt at a loss to know how to combat this denial, stigma, discrimination and secrecy. This has justified calls for 'new or different' approaches to respond to the epidemic, particularly in high-prevalence areas. Mandatory HIV case-reporting and disclosure of HIV status, particularly to sexual partners but also to communities, have been suggested as sound public health measures. Discussions have been initiated nationally, regionally and internationally on how to :

— create greater openness about HIV/AIDS among individuals and within families and communities;
— encourage more people to test for HIV, inform sexual partners about the results and prevent further infections;
— better protect people not infected from becoming infected;
— increase acceptance, care and support for people and families affected by HIV/AIDS;
— improve epidemiological surveillance of HIV and AIDS.

Vital and effective steps towards opening up the HIV/AIDS epidemic involve the encouragement of beneficial disclosure, ethical partner counselling and the appropriate use of HIV case-reporting. The UNAIDS Secretariat and WHO offer guidance concerning these issues in a context that involves commitment to human rights, ethical principles, public health and community empowerment. Such a context protects the health and safety of the individual both infected and uninfected; it also protects public health. It does so by creating an environment that encourages the most people to get tested for HIV; encourages people to change their behaviour either to prevent their own infection or that of others and, where infected, to feel able and willing to disclose their status in a way that prevents onward transmission of HIV; and results in care and compassion. Such an environment will help to open up the epidemic; reduce the denial, stigma, discrimination and secrecy surrounding HIV/AIDS; and fashion programmes that allow governments, communities and individuals to deal with the causes and consequences of HIV/AIDS in the most effective and humane ways possible.

Confidentiality is an ethical principle particularly relevant in the provision of health care.The principle of confidentiality encompasses the view that a person should be entitled to privacy with regard to his or her most personal physical and psychological secrets; but it is also the basis for an effective relationship between patient/client and health care provider, and hence the basis for the effectiveness of many public health interventions which rest on these relationships.

Only if a person feels sure that the health care provider will keep confidential any information provided will he come forward and share information that may be critical to making decisions about effective clinical care and treatment. Thus, health care professionals have long recognised and respected their duty, and the need, to protect the confidentiality of their patients. Due to the need to protect confidentiality in order to provide effective health care, health care professionals also recognise that they should normally only disclose highly personal information, such as HIV status, with the informed consent of the patient.

However, the principle of confidentiality is not absolute, and there are situations where it is not maintained. One of these occurs when necessary and relevant information is shared among health care professionals who are responsible for the clinical management of a person's health needs. Often a small group of professionals, usually in a hospital or clinic setting, will share personal information about a client, including HIV status, which is essential to the effective treatment of the case, but confidentiality will be maintained within this professional group. Another situation where confidentiality may be breached without the consent of the patient occurs when there is a clear indication that a third party may be harmed by the actions of the patient. In these situations the ethical principle of confidentiality may conflict with the ethical principle to "do no harm", and a difficult but necessary ethical weighing of the potential harms and benefits to the parties involved should be undertaken in order to decide how to proceed.

The ethical principles of confidentiality and informed consent, which have private and public health benefits, should be distinguished from secrecy which is a state of affairs often resulting from fear, shame and/or a sense of vulnerability. Whether secrecy is maintained depends solely on the personal motives of those who hold the secret. Motives to maintain secrecy in the context of HIV/AIDS involve not only fear and shame, but also denial, and fear of rejection, stigma and discrimination. To the degree that secrecy harms the infected and the uninfected, and undermines an individual's, family's or community's ability to cope positively with HIV/AIDS, it should be strongly combated.

UNAIDS and WHO are of the view that the secrecy surrounding HIV/AIDS, and the related stigma, denial and discrimination, can best be countered by a greatly increased commitment to beneficial disclosure, ethical partner counselling and appropriate use of HIV case-reporting.

PROVIDING SURVIVAL SKILLS

Providing survival skills is a vital part of HIV counselling. Knowing about survival skills helps people accept a positive HIV test result because it reinforces the message that this result does not mean the end of their life. Survival skills should be discussed in all counselling sessions, including in sessions with clients who are unaware of their HIV status and are considering being tested. Counsellors need to prepare for counselling sessions. There are, however, several things he can do to prepare himself. He needs to find out as much information as possible about HIV, AIDS, and related subjects. This information should be accurate and uptodate. He has to make himself familiar with the skills needed to prolong life and the behaviors that speed up the progression of AIDS. If he knows other people dealing with similar problems for the client, explore the client's interest in meeting these people to help in the formation of support or self-help groups.

Begin to discuss survival skills with clients as early as possible, preferably during pre-test counselling. Most people going for an HIV test are already thinking about how a positive test result may affect their life. Knowing beforehand that there are survival strategies can ease the tension. If the test does turn out to be positive, the knowledge that there is something one can do to stay healthy will help the client cope with receiving the result.

Some issues the counsellor should be aware of when he is counselling a person who intends to have an HIV test:

— Determine the reasons why the client has decided to have an HIV test. Sometimes people are pressured or coerced into having a test by another person such as a doctor, counsellor, or partner. It is important that the client, and nobody else, decides to have a test. Taking an HIV test is a big step and the client needs to be aware of the advantages and disadvantages. The test, should not be done without the client's full and genuine consent.

— Give the client accurate and uptodate information about HIV and AIDS, and correct any misconceptions the client might have. Give the client time to express any worries or fears, and address them before the test is taken.

— Stress the confidentiality of counselling and testing. It is important that the client understands that both the discussion and the results of the test will be confidential, and that nobody else will be told about them without the client's permission.

- If the client thinks that he or she might be HIV positive, you should explore the reasons. Help the client assess the risks and the effects of HIV in preparation for the results.
- Whenever possible, help the client identify a support person — a relative or a friend — to provide company when going for the test results and for post-test counselling.
- Tell the client about support groups and explore the possibility that he or she may join such a group if the HIV test is positive. This is particularly important if you sense during the interview that the client does not have a strong social support network.
- If the client has a stable sexual partner, you should explain the advantages of getting tested and getting results with the partner. Explore the difficulties and possible consequences of disclosing the test result to the partner. Try to encourage the client to bring his or her partner to a pre-test counselling session.
- Prepare the client for both a positive and a negative HIV test result. In preparation for a negative result explore with the client how to reduce his or her personal risk for HIV infection. In preparation for a positive result introduce the subjects of survival skills and positive living that will be covered in much greater detail during post-test counselling.

Survival skills are a very important subject of post-test counselling. When people find out that they are HIV positive they often feel as if their world has fallen apart and that there is no point in living any longer. Post-test counselling should help people develop coping mechanisms for dealing with their HIV status, and to realise that life is not over just because of the result of a laboratory test.

Some issues the counsellor should be aware of when he is counselling persons who have returned for their HIV test result:

— Assure that the client is ready to receive the result. You can assume that most people who have returned to the testing centre want to know their test result, but you should still ask. If you sense some hesitation, talk about the reasons. The client may not be here out of his or her own free will. Discuss the advantages and disadvantages of knowing one's HIV status. Do not give the results until you are sure the client is ready to receive them.

— Assure the client again that the result of the HIV test and the discussions of the counselling session are confidential and will not be disclosed to anyone without his or her explicit permission.

— If and when the client is ready, give the test result.

If the counsellor have just give a positive HIV test result to a client:

— Observe and assess the client's emotional state. People react in different ways to a positive result. Some people show little emotion, others react with emotional outbursts. The counsellor's role is to assist clients to deal with their emotions as they are expressed.

— Address the client's needs and concerns. This discussion must be driven by the client and not by the counsellor. This means that you should respond to the issues and topics brought up by the client, but not tell the client how he or she is feeling or what emotions he or she might be going through.

— Find out if the client has had a pre-test counselling session and what was discussed. Sometimes people are tested for HIV without pre-test counselling. In this case, you should try and cover the most important pre-test issues in the post-test counselling session.

— Discuss survival skills and strategies for positive living. These include risk reduction, nutrition, and stress management.

— Disclosure of HIV status is a very important issue at the time of post-test counselling. Explore to what extent this has been discussed during pre-test counselling. Has the client thought about whom to tell about the result? Who are the people that the client can rely on for support? Do not rush the client into making decisions about disclosure. This is a big step that has to be considered carefully.

— Remember that your main task when counselling a person who has just received a positive HIV test result is to provide emotional support and information. If you do not have the information, refer the client to another counsellor or to another source of information or support.

— After receiving a positive HIV test result, many people find it hard to concentrate on specific issues. The client's mind is racing—many points covered in the counselling session will be quickly forgotten. Encourage the client to return for further sessions of supportive counselling where issues can be dealt with, as they become important and relevant. Make a follow-up appointment.

Stress Management

Dealing with stress is an important survival skill. A person who is stressed may show the following signs and symptoms:

— social withdrawal, loss of interest in surroundings;
— moodiness, irritability, or intolerance;
— difficulty falling asleep, or early morning wakening;
— constant fatigue, difficulty in getting out of bed;
— upset stomach, loss of appetite, over-eating;
— headaches or pain in the neck and shoulders;
— loss of sexual desires or urges;
— loss of ability to concentrate;
— loss of interest in activities, apathy;

— poor performance at work or in school;
— pacing or restlessness;
— increased use of alcohol, tobacco, or other drugs.

Possible causes of stress that are related to HIV infection may be:

— receiving the result of a positive HIV test;
— involuntary disclosure of a positive HIV test;
— break-up of family or of a relationship;
— death of a spouse or child;
— financial difficulties;
— loss of employment;
— inability to talk about one's problems;
— isolation due to expected or actual stigma;
— belief that death is imminent;
— fear of dying.

A counsellor should help the clients to manage their stress:

— Encourage the clients to talk about the issues troubling them.
— Discuss potential sources of support. Sources of support can be found amongst family, relatives, friends, church groups, support groups, or counselling organisations.
— Encourage clients to rest, relax, and get enough sleep. Some people find it relaxing to pray, meditate, or to talk to themselves in private. Physical exercise is very effective for stress management. Encourage clients to take up yoga, go jogging, join an aerobics class, or go dancing.
— Encourage clients to spend time with other people and help them identify people they feel secure with:

— Try to identify the problem. It is easier to deal with stress once you know what is causing it.

— Death or sickness in the family is a common cause of stress. Another booklet in this series provides counselling guidelines for palliative care and bereavement.

— People are affected differently by stress. After a stressful event some people "shut down" and adopt a life style of mere survival without joy or expectations. Others react by becoming over-active and pushing themselves harder.

— Encourage them to adopt techniques like affirmation (I am .... I can.... I will...) and relaxation (meditation, exercise) to help them return to a pace and a style of life that is comfortable for them.

— Remember that some stress can be positive. Knowing that they are HIV positive has motivated many people to plan their lives more carefully and deliberately. They are achieving much more because they have developed a positive attitude to life.

SUPPORTING BENEFICIAL DISCLOSURE

In the context of HIV/AIDS, the term 'disclosure' refers to the act of informing any individual or organisation of the HIV status of an infected person, or it refers to the fact that such information has been transmitted, by any means, by the person him or herself, or by a third party, with or without consent. However, the purposes and the consequences of disclosure may be beneficial or harmful.

Examples of beneficial disclosure involve instances where an HIV-positive person informs a sexual partner of his status for prevention purposes, or informs family, community members or health care workers in order to share vital personal information and obtain support. Or disclosure may involve a health care worker providing information regarding an HIV/

AIDS case on a confidential basis to other health care workers involved in the management of the patient; to a health authority for surveillance purposes; or, where necessary, to a partner of an HIV-positive person to prevent onward transmission of HIV.

Examples of harmful disclosure involve cases where disclosure is made without the consent of the person who is HIV positive and has adverse consequences for that person, such as stigma, abandonment, physical violence, imprisonment, loss of job or housing, or other forms of discrimination. Harmful disclosure may also impair prevention and care activities.

Where people fear forced testing, or disclosure involving lack of confidentiality, they will avoid HIV counselling, testing, treatment and support, because these are likely to mean that their HIV status will become known against their will and they will face stigma, discrimination, lack of privacy and other negative effects. Thus, fear of lack of confidentiality and forced disclosure drives people away from HIV services, reducing opportunities to encourage and empower people to change their behaviour in order either to avoid getting infected or to avoid passing on their infection. It may also drive people away from other health care services, such as antenatal care or blood donation.

Beneficial disclosure is voluntary; respects the autonomy and dignity of the affected individuals; maintains confidentiality as appropriate; leads to beneficial results for those individuals, and for their families and sexual and drug-injecting partners; leads to greater openness in the community about HIV/AIDS; and meets the ethical imperatives of the situation where there is need to prevent onward transmission of HIV. Such beneficial disclosure, with its elements of voluntariness and confidentiality, not only maintains ethical principles but also serves a direct public health function, because it encourages people to access HIV prevention and care services. It does this by establishing a climate of trust between health care providers and those who need HIV services, allaying their fears and respecting them as people who can and will make the right decisions regarding their behaviour.

Beneficial disclosure also serves the goal of opening up the HIV/AIDS epidemic. As more people feel able and willing to disclose their status, there grows a critical mass of individuals and families within a community, and indeed within a nation, who are openly involved in dealing with the epidemic in positive and supportive ways. As a consequence, discrimination, stigma and secrecy are reduced. Nevertheless, preconditions are necessary to promote beneficial disclosure and to encourage people to access prevention and care programmes.

People must have access to voluntary counselling and testing (VCT) services in which they can learn their HIV status and receive support and referral in dealing with the news. Furthermore, they must have an incentive to find out their status such that it will mean greater social support, access to health care options and an increased ability to live a rewarding life regardless of a negative or positive status.

Up to 90 per cent of HIV-positive people in low-income countries do not know their HIV status due to the fact that there are few VCT facilities available to the populations most affected by HIV/AIDS. Even where testing is available, many people do not want to be tested because of a perception that 'nothing is to be gained' by knowing an HIV-positive status. For the poor there will be little access to HIV/AIDS treatment and care. Furthermore, there will likely be stigma and discrimination to be faced if found to be HIV positive.

However, even in resource-poor settings much can be done to improve access to voluntary counselling, HIV testing, treatment and care, though this may involve a shift of resources from "traditional" HIV programmes and activities. Primarily, there must be greater investment in establishing VCT services in communities. Secondly, incentives must be created to encourage people to undergo testing. These should take the form of community services providing support, treatment and care. Finally, disincentives to test, such as stigma and discrimination, should be removed.

There are insufficient VCT services in the communities most in need of them. More resources from national AIDS programmes should be devoted to establishing such services, which can take many forms. Most important are that VCT services are integrated into existing services where applicable (e.g. antenatal care, sexually transmitted infection (STI) clinics, family health clinics); they are user friendly (particularly to youth and women); are accessible to marginalised groups (e.g., the poor, rural populations, sex workers, drug injectors, migrants); and are designed to tie the individual using them into other support and care options (e.g., referral to STI services, support groups, family outreach programmes). The creation and availability of such services is a prerequisite if people are to learn about their HIV status and find ways of dealing with it constructively, including through disclosure.

However, the existence of VCT services is not in itself enough to get people to come forward for HIV testing. There must be incentives, and these should take the form of greater availability and affordability of care, treatment and support. In resource-poor settings, treatment, in the form of drugs, and care options are very limited. However, these obstacles can in part be overcome by innovative and far-reaching community-based programmes. Such programmes offer outreach to affected families, voluntary and confidential counselling and testing, support groups, home visits, follow-up and involvement of people living with HIV/AIDS in prevention and care activities. They may also offer models of how to 'live positively' with HIV/AIDS, through which people maximise their personal and social resources, live as best as possible in the present and plan realistically for the future. Examples of such effective community-based programmes can be found in Uganda, Tanzania and Thailand, where campaigns by non-governmental organisations (NGOs) to encourage testing have created more openness and discussion about HIV. In the parts of these countries where HIV testing has been made reasonably accessible to affected communities, the synergistic link between reducing stigma, increasing voluntary testing and encouraging disclosure has been confirmed. Each of these activities reinforces the others and leads to greater numbers of people taking advantage of voluntary counselling, testing and support. This leads to more voluntary disclosure (to spouses, lovers, family members, friends and health care providers), the adoption of low-risk behaviour and a movement towards positive living. When such programmes are well integrated into the community and are responding to its needs, they can have a profound influence on how HIV/AIDS is perceived at the individual, family and community levels.

Positive-living models, as well as the active involvement of people living with and affected by HIV/AIDS, help to change attitudes from stigma and discrimination to respect and support. Affected families and communities are able to embrace their situation, are given support in how to best deal with it, while the family member who is HIV positive is still able to contribute to family and community efforts. This helps to reduce the stigma and to change public perceptions of HIV and people living with HIV/AIDS. It also helps to encourage more people who do not know their status to come forward voluntarily for counselling and testing. Thus, greater investment needs in creating the facilities for HIV testing, as well as in backing community-based programmes which create a supportive environment and encourage people to come forward for HIV testing, counselling, care, treatment and support.

Due to considerable shame, secrecy and fear surrounding HIV, people infected with HIV are highly stigmatised. HIV is also the cause of human rights violations and acts of discrimination. As a result of the stigma and discrimination surrounding HIV/AIDS, those who do know their HIV status are afraid to disclose it because of the risk of job loss, social ostracism, violence and threats to their lives, and other adverse consequences. Those who do not know their status are afraid to get tested if they fear that the results will be made known against their will and they will face stigma and discrimination. Thus, to encourage voluntary testing, beneficial disclosure and use of HIV services, the disincentives of stigma and discrimination, and lack of confidentiality, must be removed.

Many steps can be taken to reduce stigma and discrimination. One of the most under-utilised has been public information campaigns which focus specifically on the promotion of tolerance, compassion and non-discrimination. Though the world has been inundated with public information about the fact that HIV cannot be transmitted casually, this information has not done enough to alleviate fear of HIV and AIDS and of people living with them. Public information campaigns should be conducted which involve creative, attractive, powerful messages against discrimination and stigma. Public forums on HIV/AIDS and/or community discussion groups, which focus on compassion, tolerance and support, should also be held. Where there is protection against violence and discrimination, public figures, including those living with HIV, should be involved in these public campaigns.

The involvement of people living with HIV/AIDS in public campaigns, and in policy, programmatic and community activities, is critical to give a human face to the epidemic, to reaffirm the value of people with HIV/AIDS and to change attitudes of stigma. It also ensures that policies and programmes will be sensitive to the actual needs and realities of those affected by HIV/AIDS. Other measures can be undertaken at a national level, such as the enactment of laws and policies against HIV-related discrimination and against breaches in confidentiality and informed consent.

One essential step is the training and sensitisation of professionals who work with people affected by HIV/AIDS. It is often at the hands of such professionals that people affected by HIV/AIDS suffer the worst discrimination, despite the professional and ethical responsibility to treat people who are

HIV positive with dignity and compassion, and to protect their confidentiality in appropriate ways. Key professionals who might benefit from training in nondiscrimination, confidentiality and informed consent are health care workers, police, social service providers, lawyers and judges.

Health care workers should be more empowered to handle the medical, as well as psychosocial, management of clients with HIV/AIDS. This should include training and empowerment regarding universal precautions against transmission of infectious diseases, as it is the fear of transmission of HIV among health care workers that often leads to stigma and discrimination against people with HIV/AIDS. Experience has shown that the impact of this training in health settings needs regular monitoring and staff updating to ensure that infection control procedures are maintained.

To encourage beneficial disclosure, UNAIDS and WHO recommend the following:

— Conduct public information campaigns and community forums aimed at promoting tolerance, compassion and understanding, and reducing fear, stigma and discrimination.

— Encourage participation of people living with HIV/AIDS in public information campaigns and in HIV programmes and policy formulation.

— Establish more VCT services, including in rural areas and for marginalised groups.

— Support governmental agencies, NGOs and community-based organisations (CBOs) to make community-based services, including VCT, family outreach, community support, positive living, support groups and care options more widely available.

— Encourage the media to report on HIV/AIDS in a responsible, non-discriminatory and non-sensational manner.

— Train health care workers in the management of HIV and universal precautions, in attitudes of non-discrimination, acceptance and compassion, and in the principles of confidentiality and informed consent.

— Train other professionals (social workers, police, lawyers, judges) in attitudes of non-discrimination, acceptance and compassion, and in the principles of confidentiality and informed consent.

— Train key personnel in non-health employment settings, including human resource management in industry, in promoting non-discriminatory practices in the workplace.

— Enact or reform laws, administrative guidelines and professional codes of conduct to prohibit discrimination and breaches of confidentiality related to HIV status.

— Create legal support services for those who have suffered discrimination based on HIV status.

The counsellor should be aware of the following disclosure issues when counselling for survival skills:

— People who plan to disclose their HIV status need a lot of support and emotional preparation.

— The respondents, whom clients want to disclose their HIV status to, should have correct information about HIV and AIDS, and should have an open and non-stigmatising attitude towards people living with HIV. You may need to help some clients prepare their respondents.

— Some clients may ask for your presence when disclosing their HIV status. The presence of a counsellor can support both the client and the confidante. Remember that finding out that a loved one is infected with HIV can be very stressful.

— Encourage the clients to be selective about disclosure. There are advantages and disadvantages to disclosure in each situation.

— People should never be forced or pressured to disclose their HIV status; they must only do so when they feel ready to deal with the consequences. The client and not the counsellor has to decide whom to tell and when. This may be difficult for the counsellor who may know the client's family or sexual partner.

— Talking to somebody who is HIV positive may be very helpful to a person who is considering disclosure. Some support groups of people living with HIV have trained volunteer counsellors. They have personal experience of sharing information about their HIV status and can give guidance to the client. Joining a support group and talking to other people living with HIV is always a good idea, and it is particularly helpful for reaching a decision on disclosure.

TREATMENT AND MEDICINES

There are at least 15 different types of medicines known as antiretroviral drugs (ARVs). None of these drugs can cure AIDS or eliminate HIV, but if taken in the right combination, they can slow down the progression from HIV infection to AIDS. Until recently, the drugs have been very expensive. However, an intensive international lobby has resulted in the reduction of price in some countries, and the movement is gaining ground all over Africa. ARVs are already available in specialised clinics and big hospitals in all major cities, however still at a price that places them out of reach of most of the population.

The currently available ARVs have to be taken for life. An effective treatment requires that at least three different drugs are taken at the same time. The drugs have major, and sometimes life-threatening side-effects. In countries where these drugs have been available for a long time, about one in three persons stops taking them because of side effects or inability to follow the very strict drug regimen. There are a number of other medicines that are known to be beneficial to people living with HIV through their action of preventing common opportunistic infections. These are generally much more affordable and more widely available than ARVs.

A counsellor should be aware of the types of medical treatment available to people living with HIV in the community, and how to access these treatments. However, it is not wise to discuss medical therapies with the client unless expertise in this area. There are, however, alternate therapies being explored by PLWHA groups all over the world, whether they have access to ARV treatment or not. Many of these therapies have proven beneficial. The counsellor should explore among local support groups what types of natural or alternative medicines are available. The main guidelines in recommending alternative therapies are that the counsellor should not believe any claims of a "cure" of AIDS; the treatment should not do any harm to the patient; and it should not waste the patient's money without providing any benefit.

Taking vitamin supplements, improved nutrition, prevention and early treatment of minor infections and avoiding stress can help prolong the client's life. Prompt attention to minor aches, pains, skin rashes, or injuries is essential for health and survival.

Here are some alternative therapies that PLWHAs have found useful. Remember that therapies such as aromatherapy, herbal remedies, reflexology, and hypnotherapy require a qualified practitioner:

meditation	the process of relaxing daily in a quiet setting to focus deeply on body energy and breathing techniques;
relaxation	taking a short break away from work or chores to rest and control your breathing and body's response to increased tension;

(Contd...)

(Contd...)

massage	kneading or rubbing parts of the body to promote circulation, suppleness, pain relief or relaxation;
aromatherapy	the application of fragrant essential oils to relieve tension and certain minor ailments;
herbal remedies	the treatment of ailments with plants. There are many effective and widely known herbal remedies for common ailments such as diarrhoea. Some herbal remedies, for instance the African potato, are believed to boost the immune system and help fight off infections;
reflexology	a form of therapy Where pressure is applied to specific areas on the feet and hands, which stimulate the blood supply and nerves to create a relaxing and healing effect on other body parts;
art therapy	drawing, painting or other forms of art as a way of relaxing or expressing emotions;
hypnotherapy	inducing a state of deep relaxation and concentration in which deeper parts of the mind are accessible for the treatment of emotional problems.
	Remind the client to "listen to your body". If eating in a certain way or receiving a certain type of treatment makes the client feel better, it will almost certainly be beneficial.

NUTRITIONAL NEEDS

Good nutrition is the only form of therapy that is available to most people. It is generally affordable because unrefined and unprocessed foods tend to be cheaper, though healthier. Nutrition as a therapy can improve the quality of life for people living with HIV because it can help them feel in charge. It allows them to do something practical to help themselves. People living with HIV need to protect their immune system because it is weakened by the HIV infection. They can do this by paying attention to two rules:

i) Do not give your immune system other things to fight. You are most vulnerable to the effects of HIV when your body is trying to fight off other types of infections or when it is weakened by stress or exhaustion.

ii) Strengthen your immune system by providing your body with the necessary nutrients to remain strong. This means eating a healthy and balanced diet.

A counsellor should become familiar with the rules for healthy eating in order to advise the clients.

When foods are "refined" it means that all the goodness has been removed. When foods have been "processed" it means things like colourings and preservatives — which can be harmful to the health — have been added.

A healthy plate should look like this:

— *Whole Grain (50%):* Grains should be whole, even if ground for thick porridge. For example, sorghum, millet, whole ground maize, whole wheat bread made from whole wheat flour, brown (unpolished) rice, barley, oat porridge, brekweet, or maltabella.

— *Vegetables (30%):* Combine yellow (pumpkin, butternut, carrots, and sweet potato) with white (onions, leeks, cabbage, cauliflower) and green vegetables (spinach, rape, broccoli, okra, pumpkin leaves). Eat lots of vegetables everyday.

— *Pulses (750)*: Pulses should make up the majority of protein in the diet: lentils, peas, nuts, dry bears, peanut butter, chick peas, beans, and soya (soya mince or TVP). Soya and round nuts are "perfect proteins". Just like meat all the others must be combined with whole grains to make 100% protein.

— *Side Dish (5%):* This group should make up no more than 5 per cent of the total amount eaten. It includes:

fruits: eat when fresh and when in season. Avocados, tomatoes and peppers are also in this group.

meat: little or no meat is recommended. Fish and chicken are best. If meat is desired, eat liver, kidney, or heart as they are high in iron.

dairy: milk, cheese and milk products should be eaten very sparingly. Don't eat any dairy at all when you have diarrhoea, except yoghurt and lacto, which are good at all times. Eggs are good occasionally.

Vitamins and minerals are natural substances contained in food which are needed by the body in very small quantities for many different functions, including boosting the immune system. They are called micro-nutrients.

Many people living with HIV take additional micro-nutrients in the form of tablets. But remember, vitamin tablets are no replacement for a healthy diet. If the client is poor, do not recommend spending money on vitamin preparations. The priority should be a balanced nutrition for the family. If there is money left over, then the client may consider vitamin supplements.

One combination recommended by PLWHA groups consists of zinc, vitamins A, C, and E and selenium (ZACES). ZACES is an infection fighting combination of vitamins and minerals. It increases the body's natural resistance and protects against the side effects of medications.

Zinc	1 x 10mg tablet, twice daily
Vitamin A	1 x 25,000 I.U. tablet, once daily
Vitamin C	2 x 500mg tablet twice daily (or 4 x 250mg twice daily)
Selenium	1 x 100mcg tablet daily (or 2 × 50 mgtwice daily)
Medox	12 × 12 1 tablet daily
Garlic	Up to 5 cloves a day

Foods to avoid include:

— Sugar and all foods containing sugar: this includes cool drinks, cakes, sweets and cookies.

-- Tinned, processed and refined foods.

— *Strong tea and coffee*: rooibos tea, herb tea, fruit tea, bush tea and decaffeinated coffee can be good substitutes.

— Alcohol and tobacco.

— *Red meat and pork*: liver and kidney are best if you crave red meat.

— *Cooking oil*: except olive oil or cold pressed oils. Heating oil to cook with it destroys any goodness. Use it for salads only. Fats (dairy products) should be used sparingly and not at all when you have diarrhoea.

Health to achieve long-term survival with HIV can be compared to a table with four legs representing mental, physical, spiritual, and social health. The top of the table is nutrition.

i) *Mental:* Encourage the clients to learn to co-exist with the virus. By giving the clients accurate and positive information about HIV and the immune system, you can help them adapt their lifestyle to overcome the immediate threats of HIV infection and to adopt a mental state in which they are not always feeling fragile and in danger.

ii) *Spiritual:* Encourage the clients to seek spiritual support, whatever their religious and cultural background. Prayer or meditation can induce deep mental and spiritual relaxation and renewal.

iii) *Physical:* Encourage the clients to learn the practical steps they can take to improve and maintain health, e.g., exercising.

iv) *Social:* Encourage the clients to join a support group and to become active in the community. Social isolation because of fear of being rejected or because of past experiences of rejection is bad for the clients' health and survival.

MAINTAINING SEXUAL HEALTH

After receiving the result of a positive HIV test, some people feel 'off' sex, some feel dirty or 'contaminated', and some believe that they can no longer have normal sexual relations. Yet a person living with HIV has the same sexual feelings and needs as anyone else, and there is no reason why these should be denied. Counsellors can help people understand this. At the same time they must make their clients aware of the risks so they can make informed and responsible choices about their sexual and reproductive lives.

The counsellor should be able to talk to the clients freely and objectively about sex. Condom use is a key issue to be discussed. The counsellor have to impress on his clients that consistent use of a male or female condom in every act of sexual intercourse is important for their own health and the health of their partners. If the partner is not infected, then he or she risks becoming infected with HIV. If the partner is already HIV positive, then both partners risk re-infecting each other, and thereby increasing the number of virus particles in their system. This may result in a faster progression of the HIV infection to AIDS. Therefore, strict condom use or practising non-penetrative sex will protect both partners, whatever their status. Other important counselling issues related to reproductive and sexual health include:

— family planning;
— abstinence;
— partner notification;
— sexually transmitted diseases;
— changes in the menstrual cycle;
— transmission of HIV from mother to child.

Role of a counsellor is to:

— provide accurate and relevant information so that the client can make informed choices;
— give and explore options; recognise and respect the uniqueness of the client; be aware of one's own beliefs and values;
— know when to refer the client to another counsellor or agency for more appropriate and accurate information.

The clients may be concerned about whether or not they can have children. The counsellor need to advise them on the risks of HIV transmission to the child. Most of the transmission occurs during labour or through breast-feeding. However, most children born to HIV positive mothers are not infected with HIV, and there are interventions that can reduce the risk of HIV transmission to the infant.

HIV positive women who wish to conceive should seek out good ante-natal and obstetric care. After delivery, they should avoid breast-feeding or practise "safer breast-feeding". The four components of safer breast-feeding are:

— exclusive breast-feeding for up to six months;
— condom use during the lactation period;

— proper positioning and attachment of the baby during every feed; and
— immediate medical attention for minor infections of the breast or lesions in the baby's mouth.

PROMOTING HIV CASE-REPORTING

HIV case-reporting has been promoted as a means to open up the HIV/AIDS epidemic; decrease denial; improve access to prevention and care services for those affected by HIV/AIDS; and obtain more accurate information on the prevalence and incidence of HIV and AIDS for surveillance purposes. Under such a policy, health care providers would be required to report by name all HIV cases diagnosed by them to a health authority. Other forms of case-reporting involve the use of a code, sometimes called a "unique identifier", for each case; or provide information on cases anonymously.

While AIDS case-reporting has been implemented in most countries, implementation of HIV case-reporting has been much more limited. Many countries started to collect information on HIV cases at the beginning of the epidemic but later dropped the practice when the infection became widespread. The reasons were the high cost and complexity of maintaining the system, the lack of effective treatment or preventive options once people were discovered to be HIV positive, and the small additional benefit for surveillance purposes.

However, there has been a recent trend in high-income countries to employ HIV, as well as AIDS, case-reporting. This trend is based on the fact that, where antiretroviral therapies are available, the access to, and use of, these drugs has dramatically decreased the incidence of AIDS. As a result, AIDS cases are no longer an accurate base for calculating back to HIV incidence and prevalence. Furthermore, in these countries, case-reporting of HIV helps to monitor the access of those who are HIV positive to appropriate services and treatment, including the use of anti-retrovirals. However, neither the reporting of HIV cases nor the reporting of AIDS cases has been useful in low-income countries. For surveillance purposes, data collected on the basis of case-reporting of HIV or AIDS have been problematic.

In general, HIV/AIDS surveillance involves the routine collection, analysis and dissemination of accurate epidemiological information regarding the spread and distribution of HIV infection. Surveillance is an essential part of the response to the epidemic entailing a number of important objectives:

— to monitor trends in prevalence and incidence of HIV in populations;
— to assess disease burden in terms of morbidity and mortality due to HIV/AIDS;
— to be able to plan HIV prevention and care programmes directed at the particular epidemiological situation;
— to provide data for estimates and projections of the number of people with HIV/AIDS and AIDS-related mortality;
— to monitor the impact of the national response to the HIV/AIDS epidemic;
— to reinforce commitment to AIDS prevention and care through awareness of the numbers affected and their needs.

But the data obtained from HIV and AIDS case-reporting in many countries have not been useful for the stated objectives of surveillance largely for the following reasons.

— Less than 10 per cent of HIV-positive people have been tested for HIV, so most are unaware of their status.
— Many people do not want to know their status, given the stigma and discrimination attached to a positive result and the fact that they will not have access to treatment or care.

— Among health care providers, there are problems with under-diagnosis and underreporting of HIV and AIDS cases, including the fact that health care providers may be reluctant to report cases by name for reasons of confidentiality and privacy.

— In contrast, where the information is provided anonymously to avoid breaches in confidentiality, there is potential for multiple reporting of the same case.

— There is insufficient capacity and infrastructure to maintain confidentiality for either named or coded reporting, which further deters people presenting for tests. These conditions make HIV case-reporting in resource-poor countries unreliable.

Advocates of HIV case-reporting point to potential benefits in terms of prevention and increased access to care. However, reporting HIV cases to health authorities does not necessarily lead to any additional benefit for either the client or the community, and may divert resources from more effective prevention and care strategies. Thus, where resources are limited, the appropriate balance must be found in the use of various prevention and care strategies that have different levels of costs and impact.

Strategies such as public information campaigns, youth education and distribution of condoms are relatively cost-effective ways of reaching large numbers of people for prevention and care purposes. Case-reporting, however, is expensive, and does not increase access to prevention and care services in itself. To be effective in prevention and care terms, case-reporting must be meaningfully integrated into a host of HIV-related services, such as VCT, health and social support services for those HIV positive and/or presenting with AIDS-related illnesses, and greater access to HIV-related drugs and treatments. Resources should be put into developing these services before they are significantly diverted to case-reporting.

In light of these concerns, UNAIDS and WHO recommend HIV case-reporting only where certain conditions exist. These are:

— widespread access to, and use of, HIV testing;
— protection against breaches of confidentiality so as not to deter testing and reporting;
— access to effective care, including anti-retrovirals;
— capacity within the health system to collect accurate data, and to compile, analyse, and act upon them, including follow-up of cases.

SUPPORTIVE COUNSELLING

Supportive counselling may be centre-based—the client coming to see the counsellor when they need advice and support. Or it may be home-based. The advantage of home-based supportive counselling is that clients may be seen in their own environment. It may not be very expensive if it is well planned, because several clients can often be seen in one visit. It is an opportunity to get to know clients better, to know their social and material situation, and to get to know their families and support networks. Examples of supportive counselling activities include:

— setting up tasks or goals (remember to check or follow up on goals on next visit or session);
— providing a "sounding board" (being a listener) for clients to express their concerns or talk about particular issues;
— working with the family, e.g., to improve the client's social support, or to help create more openness within the family;
— helping clients to improve their communication skills, especially if they are preparing to disclose their HIV status.

There are limitations to remember:

— Supportive home-based counselling requires a lot of resources.

— A long-lasting supportive counselling relationship may create material and emotional dependency on the counsellor.

— Some clients may feel that their privacy is being invaded by the counsellor.

— A counsellor may become too involved with a small number of clients, which will reduce overall effectiveness in job.

— Supportive counselling often involves repetition of things that have been discussed before. Clients who are stressed or upset will not absorb information the first time they hear it because of their emotional state. Be patient and be prepared to repeat discussions and to restate important messages several times.

PEER COUNSELLING

Peer counselling overcomes barriers caused by class, age, gender, sexual orientation, or HIV status. Peer counsellors have similar characteristics and experiences as their clients.

In peer counselling it is important to remember the following:

Do	*Do Not*
establish ground rules	judge or penalise
respect individuality	take over the burden
acknowledge the limitations of counsellors	argue
refer when stuck	ignore
listen	instruct

The advantages of peer counselling are that:

— it is easier for the client to feel at ease with a counsellor and the discussion will therefore be more open and free;

— most barriers and boundaries between counsellor and client are removed, e.g., language, age, gender, etc.; the sessions are informal and tend to be more spontaneous;

— the counsellor and the client frequent the same social circles and often live or work in proximity. This makes the counselling sessions more accessible and often more affordable for the client;

— the peer counsellor may provide a role model for the client that is easy to emulate; counselling may be linked to group support if several peers meet together.

The disadvantages of peer counselling are that:

— knowledge may be limited within the peer group so there may be misinformation and misconceptions;

— confidentiality may be compromised by the informal nature of the interactions;

— dependency on the counsellor may develop because of the easy access and the frequent social contact; there may be tendencies to compete within peer groups;

— problems of some clients may be trivialised as everybody in the peer group may face similar hardships.

REFERENCES

Eastwood, A., and A. Maynard. 1988. Treating AIDS Patients: Is it Ethical to be Efficient" Paper presented at the First International Conference on the Global Impact of AIDS, London, March.

Egal F. Valstar A., *HIV/AIDS and nutrition: helping families and communities to cope*, Rome: Food and Agriculture Organisation, 2000.

EngenderHealth, *STI/HIV Prevention – Quick Reference Cards for Health Care Providers – What Every Client Should Know*, New York, 2001.

Institute of Medicine, National Academy of Sciences, *Mobilising Against AIDS*, Cambridge, Mass.: Harvard University Press, 1986.

South African AIDS Training (SAT) Programme, *Counselling Guidlines on Survival Skills for People Living with HIV*, 2001.

UNAIDS, *Report on the global HIV/AIDS Epidemic*, 2002.

Welbourn, A., "Stepping Stones: A Training Package on HIV/AIDS, communication and relationship skills", *Strategies for Hope*, 1995.

7

Monitoring HIV/AIDS Care

The HIV epidemic first appeared as a range of opportunistic infections and other diseases defining AIDS, and the counting of new AIDS diagnoses became a central component of HIV/ AIDS surveillance systems. However, there were several important limitations. First, AIDS counts provided little information about current patterns of HIV transmission because they represented infections acquired years in the past. Second, AIDS diagnosis required clinical and laboratory expertise that was absent in many countries, particularly those of the developing world. Third, AIDS counting suffered from the limitation that health care workers did not accord a high priority to the passive reporting of cases. On the other hand, AIDS reporting did have the potential to graphically demonstrate the impact of HIV infection in terms of advanced illness, even if it was restricted in most countries to the first episode of illness that satisfied the AIDS case definition.

The advent of the HIV antibody test in 1985 opened up the possibility of directly measuring the prevalence or incidence of infection in populations. Countries from different part of the world came up with a variety of approaches to monitoring HIV prevalence. Some countries relied on routine voluntary HIV testing as a means of monitoring prevalence while other countries established comprehensive systems that involved sampling a wide range of population groups at regular intervals. In a third group of countries, prevalence was measured through occasional surveys that were implemented as resources and necessity dictated.

The World Health Organisation recommended that measurement of HIV prevalence be done using the anonymous unlinked approach which was designed to minimise the selection bias associated with voluntary testing and to protect the confidentiality of participants. Methods for serological surveillance were greatly refined in the era of HIV infection with the conduct of large-scale regular surveys in a wide variety of populations.

Monitoring of the other STDs was generally not well done since the diagnosis usually required a genital examination making special surveys expensive and logistically difficult. Furthermore, STD reporting was even more prone to underdiagnosis and underreporting than AIDS reporting since many people with STDs are asymptomatic or obtain treatment through pharmacies or other venues that do not report cases. Therefore, most countries have relied on some form of passive surveillance system for STDs.

Despite these major challenges, most countries now accept the need to monitor HIV and AIDS in a manner that is epidemiologically valid and respects confidentiality. In virtually every country, systems have been established for AIDS case reporting and in most countries the prevalence of HIV has been reasonably well characterised among the higher risk populations.

ISSUES OF SURVEILLANCE

The role of surveillance is to provide information to support the development and assessment of health programmes. In some countries, there is ongoing confusion about the role of surveillance. In particular, there remains a view in some sectors that one of the roles of surveillance is to detect people with HIV infection for the purpose of subjecting them to direct intervention of some kind, sometimes even involving law enforcement activities.

HIV sentinel surveillance does not require special procedures or methodologies. However, there are some specific issues that should be taken into consideration in implementing HIV sentinel surveillance. Implementation of HIV sentinel surveillance will require a careful selection of sentinel groups, based on their relevance to the epidemic, their accessibility and the feasibility of the study.

Traditionally, the recommended groups for HIV sentinel surveillance were STD patients (high-risk behaviours) and antenatal clinic attenders (low risk or as a proxy of the general population). In addition, data could be available from blood donors and limited serosurveys in sex workers. This methodology was developed looking primarily at the African epidemic and the reality of the African countries, where STD patients are readily available in most health facilities and antenatal screening for syphilis the commonest test for pregnant women.

In several Asian countries, STD patients are rarely seen in the public health facilities. For confidentiality or other reasons, they seek treatment at private practices or prefer to try self-medication. The small numbers and the implicit selection bias make them a difficult group to monitor for HIV surveillance. In addition, antenatal clinic care does not usually include a syphilis test at the first visit (probably due to the low prevalence of syphilis). When blood is collected from pregnant women, it is usually only a small drop for hemoglobin evaluation. This makes unlinked anonymous testing in this group extremely difficult.

On the other hand, sex workers, who are mostly floating and difficult to access in Africa, are often organised in well established brothels or massage parlours. In this setting, HIV sentinel surveillance can be easily implemented if blood is regularly taken for screening of other diseases, e.g., syphilis. Military recruits have also been used successfully in Thailand to monitor the HIV epidemic. Migrant workers, sailors and fishermen can also be considered for HIV surveillance in specific situations. Blood donors remain a useful sentinel group in most populations that have universal HIV screening programmes.

Appropriate analysis of HIV sentinel surveillance data requires the calculation of confidence intervals around the prevalence estimate. Confidence intervals are essential statistical measures of error and should be included in the analysis and reports of HIV sentinel surveillance. Finding them in surveillance report is however the exception rather than the rule. Attempts should be made to be more scientific and clearly indicate in presenting results of HIV sentinel surveillance both the relevance and the limitations of the data.

Data available from several Asian countries, including the Philippines, Indonesia, Bangladesh and, China, show HIV prevalence rates increasing very slowly, even in high-risk behaviour groups such as sex workers. This contrasts with the exponential increase seen in other populations. Several reasons have been proposed for this pattern, including the relatively low intensity of risk behaviours, particularly commercial sex. Under these circumstances, analysing these trends poses a special challenge to the surveillance system because HIV sentinel surveillance can only detect relatively marked increases in prevalence in a short period of time.

For meaningful interpretation, results of sentinel surveillance cannot be aggregated between different sites, except under the very unusual circumstance where it can be assumed with confidence that the sites draw from populations uniformly affected. Since this is rare, it is not recommended that data from separate sentinel sites be aggregated. Prevalence rates should be calculated separately per site and sentinel group. If a summary statistic is required, the most appropriate would be a median value with range of rates, or a confidence interval, for any given type of sentinel site.

Incidence Monitoring

Of central importance in targeting or assessing prevention activity is the rate at which new HIV infection is occurring, or the incidence. Apart from direct measurement through longitudinal surveys, which are expensive and difficult to sustain, HIV incidence can be estimated from back-projection of AIDS cases, or from repeat cross-sectional surveys.

At present, few countries are attempting to regularly and systematically estimate HIV incidence using one or more of the available methods. Although some expertise in modelling and statistics is available in many countries, it is often underutilised in the estimation of HIV incidence. Another measure of HIV incidence can be obtained through the monitoring of HIV prevalence in young age groups.

Monitoring Advanced Manifestations of HIV Infection

A good understanding of the spectrum of advanced HIV disease is essential for the planning of support and care services, and for assessing the benefit over time of new therapeutic and prophylactic agents. Monitoring of disease spectrum need not take place on any wide scale; it is more practical to select a small number of experienced clinical sites, to regularly report on advanced treatment manifestations, and patterns or therapy.

Monitoring of Prevalence and Incidence of Other STDs

Considerable thought and effort must continue to go into the design of surveillance systems for the other STDs. For too long, methods that were clearly developed for other infectious diseases have been uncritically used for STD surveillance, with the consequence that there is little in the way of reliable estimates of the incidence and prevalence of most STDs, and the extent of morbidity that they actually cause. In addition, innovative ways must be developed to include cases that are treated in venues that often do not report to public health authorities, such as private physicians and pharmacies.

Surveillance of HIV in Children

Given the number of women affected by HIV in developing countries, the potential for vertical transmission to newborn children is significant. Although the number of children infected by this route is unknown, the numbers are likely small at present compared to adult infections. However, HIV infections in newborns have an importance that far outweighs their numerical value because they are potentially preventable.

Programmes that offer voluntary HIV counselling and testing to pregnant women and appropriate therapy to those infected are needed to prevent vertical transmission of HIV to newborns. In this regard, the surveillance of HIV in children is important since it can help to define the need for such programmes, guide their implementation, and evaluate their effectiveness. Surveillance of HIV infection in early childhood and adolescence is also deficient. The first opportunity surveillance systems have to observe the emergence of HIV infection in this population is when girls become pregnant and attend antenatal clinics, or when boys are enrolled in the military.

By the age of 15—the earliest age included in routine surveillance in most countries—some boys and girls may have already become infected with HIV, as found in Manipur state in India, Cambodia and Thailand. Surveillance systems should become more sensitive to age and sex differentials in young people.

Behavioural Surveillance

Perhaps more so than any other continent, Asian countries are experiencing highly varied HIV epidemics, which are due to a number of factors including differential levels of risk behaviours such as multiple sexual partnerships and injecting drug use. Additionally, because Asia consists of both developing and developed countries with a variety of religious and cultural backgrounds, these risk behaviours are situated in highly varied socioeconomic and cultural environments that can either help or hinder the spread of HIV.

For example, the widespread epidemics in Thailand and Cambodia are based on the high patronage of commercial sex workers in those countries by males. Vietnam, on the other hand, has to date experienced a predominantly IDU-associated HIV epidemic, with concern growing that significant heterosexual spread will occur as well. Although HIV and AIDS case reports are still moderate for Papua New Guinea, that country is expected to face the prospect of a rapidly expanding HIV epidemic because of high rates of multiple sexual partnerships that are not commercially based.

A growing number of Asian countries such as Thailand, the Philippines, Indonesia, India, and Cambodia have initiated behavioural surveillance surveys (BSS) to understand the role of and track behavioural risks for HIV. BSS has its roots in HIV and STD surveillance and takes these methodologic concepts to the monitoring of HIV risk behaviours.

HIV prevalence taken from HIV surveillance is indicative of sexual behaviours from several years back and is slow to change even when risk behaviours may be changing rapidly. BSS thus bring surveillance data closer to what prevention programs require by providing systematic measurements of risk behaviours over time.

Given the emerging epidemics, countries should be seriously considering adding behavioural surveillance to their epidemic monitoring efforts. Specifically, while existing BSS projects have concentrated on sex workers and various occupational sub-groups of males that tend to visit sex workers, efforts are needed to conduct behavioural surveillance in areas where injecting drug users and men who have sex with men are located in sizable numbers.

Researchers have struggled with determining the important risk behaviors to track and how to best measure them. Consensus is beginning to form around five types of behaviors and characteristics that help to predict the course of the epidemic:

i) Age at first intercourse
ii) Type of sex partners (e.g., casual, commercial)

iii) Number of sex partners by type
iv) Condom use
v) Needle-sharing (for injection drug user surveys)
vi) Other factors affecting risk taking, such as alcohol and substance use

Such behaviors are sensitive and respondents may be reluctant to discuss them openly. Surveys thus require well-trained interviewers and appropriate interview settings. Behavioral surveillance, like other surveys reliant on self-reports, must be carefully implemented and validated through other data since self-reported behavioural data can be biased.

Behavioral surveillance is not a panacea for understanding all facets of HIV risk behaviors. In fact, it should be limited to only a few key target groups with a survey instrument containing rapport-building questions and a small but carefully chosen set of risk behavioral questions.

Indepth information about target groups, the evaluation of specific interventions, and relationships between several behavioral variables are better obtained through quantitative and qualitative behavioral research specifically designed to answer these questions. They are necessary adjuncts to behavioral surveillance that together form a comprehensive package of monitoring and evaluation. For example, sexual networking patterns play an important role in the rapidity with which HIV is spread within special populations (e.g., sex workers, clients of sex workers or highly mobile populations, etc.) and within broader segments of the society (e.g., women without sexual risk behaviour). These patterns can be monitored to some extent through the application of behavioral surveillance, but also require other types of socio-behavioral investigations (e.g., qualitative/ ethnographic studies).

There is a need to develop minimum common approaches and methodologies for STD surveillance as well. Given the well-documented link between STD and HIV transmission, it is critical to assess how STD rates are affecting the course of AIDS epidemics. With a few notable exceptions, there is a poor understanding of STD prevalence in countries. Analysed together, HIV, STD, and behavioral surveillance can provide complementary data to understand and track different facets of sexually transmitted diseases and their risk behaviours.

Monitoring HIV Testing Policies and Programs

HIV testing may serve any of the following objectives:

i) *Screening*: To ensure safe blood transfusion and organ transplant through screening of blood and blood products, and of tissues, sperm or ova from donors.

ii) *Surveillance*: Unlinked and/or anonymous testing of serum (or other body fluids) for the purpose of monitoring HIV prevalence over time in a given population.

iii) *Diagnosis of HIV infection*: Voluntary testing in order to inform individuals about their serostatus.

HIV testing policies and programmes are relevant to the monitoring of HIV/AIDS epidemics regardless of the original objective for testing, the test results unlinked from identifying information may be used additionally for surveillance. For example, test results from blood donors and those seeking diagnosis are often used in surveillance reports.

Testing strategies vary widely and the appropriate test or combination of tests depend on three criteria:

i) the objective of the test (for screening, surveillance, or diagnosis);

ii) the sensitivity and specificity of the test(s) being used; and

iii) the prevalence of HIV infection in the population being tested.

Most HIV tests detect HIV antibody in serum/plasma or other body fluids. Although HIV antibody testing has been available since 1985, tests have recently become available to detect viral antigen. These are much more expensive than HIV antibody tests and are used by only a few Asian and Pacific countries, generally only in specialised medical settings. Tests that detect antibody in fluids such as saliva or urine, although available, are presently only used for research purposes. These collection methods and tests have great potential for use in surveillance testing as they will help reduce some logistical difficulties and cost.

Tests commonly used in developing countries are based on the presence of HIV antibody in serum/ plasma, i.e., ELISA, Western Blot, rapid tests. In most countries, testing strategies consist of an initial screening test, usually an ELISA-based test, followed (for reactive specimens only) with a second (supplemental) test, generally either a second ELISA and/or Western Blot test.

Testing strategies vary tremendously across countries and within each broad objective (screening, surveillance, and diagnosis). Complex technical, programmatic and ethical/human rights issues abound. The issues presented below are crosscutting and are encountered in most developing countries.

Financial and qualified human resources are insufficient in most countries to provide adequate coverage for quality blood screening, surveillance, and diagnostic testing. Policy makers must carefully evaluate and provide guidelines for HIV testing options that are appropriate to the country, the purpose of testing and are affordable. Resources must be allocated for surveillance, blood screening and diagnosis, while carefully balancing these needs within the larger public health needs. Innovative approaches must be considered for tapping additional resources, such as referring testing clients to the community for counselling services; also, there is a need to increase and improve training at all levels.

There is an urgent need to assure quality throughout the testing process to ensure accurate results and confidence in data and results. This can be achieved by developing standard procedures, increasing and improving training for field workers (data collectors) and lab technicians, and monitoring the entire process.

HIV testing has the potential for human rights abuses, including marginalisation, coercion, discrimination and violence. Policy makers should develop and enforce clear policies on confidentiality and the use of test results and include persons living with HIV/AIDS in policy formulation. Legal provisions must be established to protect testing clients from abuse. Once these policies are developed, they must be disseminated and included in training for all people involved in the testing process from the point of first contact in health care settings, to the lab technicians to the counsellors.

There is an increasing demand for early diagnosis of HIV infection, both for personal knowledge and decision making and for medical management. Testing should always be accompanied by counselling, support services and treatment when available. Before aggressive case finding for medical management can be recommended, policy makers must consider the availability of treatment options and balance resource allocations of the overall public health program. Clear policies regarding use of test results and confidentiality must be established and enforced.

A number of developing countries are considering the use of HIV Rapid Tests for home-based testing. Policy makers should carefully consider the complexity of the administration and interpretation of the tests and the wide ranging implications and effects home testing can have, including the psychosocial support requirements and opportunities for human rights abuses. These must be weighed against the potential benefits and be guided by clear regulation of the use of HIV tests outside of the laboratory setting.

MONITORING HIV/AIDS CARE AND SUPPORT PROGRAMMES

People living with HIV/AIDS require a wide range of services, including psychological, social, legal and clinical ones. Care and support programmes must therefore be developed to respond to these needs and demands. Complicating the situation, these needs reflect an environment in both industrialised and resource-constrained settings in which stigma, discrimination, fear, neglect and impoverishment surround HIV/AIDS to various degrees in the community, workplaces and health care settings. To address these needs, HIV/AIDS care and support programmes should have the objectives of:

i) ensuring equitable access to diagnosis, health care, pharmaceuticals and comprehensive supportive services;
ii) reducing morbidity and mortality from HIV/AIDS and related complications;
iii) promoting opportunities for preventing HIV transmission within the delivery of care and support services; and
iv) improving the quality of life of both adults and children living with HIV/AIDS and their families.

Providing care to people living with HIV/AIDS and to their families requires a broad range of services that include not only clinical care focusing on diagnosis and treatment but also supportive and complementary services to ensure that adequate nutrition, psychological, social and daily living support are available. Efforts to prevent HIV transmission also need to be strengthened whenever opportunities arise.

Comprehensive HIV/AIDS care must include:

i) clinical care for everyone,
ii) psychological support,
iii) socioeconomic support,
iv) involvement of people living with HIV/AIDS and their families and
v) respect for human rights and legal needs.

Clinical care for everyone: Everyone should receive clinical care regardless of gender and age. Services include counselling and testing for diagnostic purposes; prophylaxis of opportunistic infections; management of HIV/AIDS-related illnesses; control of tuberculosis and management of sexually transmitted infections; management of HIV disease with antiretroviral combination therapy; palliative care; access to drugs related to HIV/AIDS, including drugs for opportunistic infections, cancer related to HIV/AIDS and anti-retroviral drugs; interventions to reduce the mother-to-child transmission of HIV; support systems such as functioning laboratories and drug management systems; nutritional support; health education measures; adequate universal precautions in clinical settings; and postexposure prophylaxis.

Psychological support: Psychological support includes initial and follow-up counselling services to meet the emotional and spiritual needs of people living with HIV/AIDS and their families and to assist in disclosure, including psychosocial support through support groups and other peer, volunteer or outreach approaches within communities.

Socioeconomic support: Material and social support is needed within communities to ensure that nutritional and daily living needs are met. Various options include microcredit schemes; housing; food support; helping hands in the household; health insurance schemes that include HIV/AIDS care and treatment; and planning and support for orphans and vulnerable children in households and communities.

Involvement of people living with HIV/AIDS and their families: People need to be involved in the planning and delivery of comprehensive care to ensure that HIV/AIDS care, treatment and support programmes intended for them address their needs, reinforce adherence, prevention and care, promote health-seeking behaviour and respect their human rights. Respect for human rights and legal needs. Services are needed that address stigma and discrimination in health facilities, in communities and in the workplace and promote equal access to care. This should also include succession planning and protection of property.

All strategic plans of national AIDS programmes should reflect this comprehensive approach to HIV/AIDS care, which should be promoted by public and nongovernmental health programmes and institutions. "Each service in this comprehensive approach reinforces and is linked to other services in a continuum of care that begins when a person learns of his or her HIV status and is offered for the duration of the illness comprehensive care and support that also addresses the holistic needs of people living with HIV/AIDS and their family members."

Access to comprehensive care should include access to antiretroviral combination therapy. It is well established that sustained use of anti-retroviral drugs increases survival, improves the quality of life, reduces hospitalisation and morbidity and mitigates socioeconomic impact. Care and antiretroviral combination therapy have also been documented to begin to alleviate stigma and fear.

Decreasing prices and international support to mobilise resources to purchase these drugs is beginning to ensure access for those in need. Efforts to increase access by international organisations such as WHO and UNICEF also contribute to increasing access to care. As prices are reduced, countries negotiate with the pharmaceutical industry and standardised guidelines are developed, countries will increasingly be able to scale up access beyond the current few demonstration and referral sites.

To enable people seeking care to determine their serostatus and to access relevant HIV/AIDS care, treatment and support services, all opportunities should be used to promote HIV testing and counselling within general outpatient and inpatient services, tuberculosis and sexually transmitted infection programmes, community health services, workplace clinics and any other site where resources allow. Upon diagnosis, counselling and HIV/AIDS care needs should be established and follow-up referral to comprehensive care must be ensured.

Multiple providers or various programmes often offer the range of HIV/AIDS care, treatment and support services, although some programmes offer a wide range of comprehensive services within one site. Partnerships and collaboration between all the various providers are therefore essential to enable timely access to appropriate services. The HIV/AIDS care continuum illustrates how these links should function in a referral system in which care providers at any service point know who provides other services, where these services are located and when and how to make a referral.

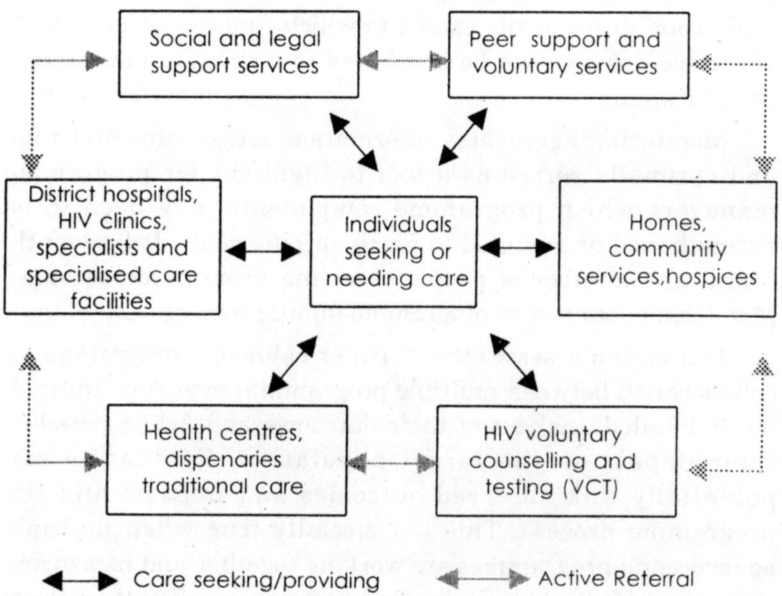

Figure 1. The HIV/AIDS Care Continuum

Monitoring and Evaluation System

As international efforts to increase access to health care, pharmaceuticals and supportive services for people living with HIV/AIDS and their families are strengthened, the need for information on monitoring and evaluation also grows. Care and support indicators are intended to provide information for local, national and international programmes on key trends in the delivery of HIV/AIDS services. The information required to measure progress can be drawn from data from such sources as national surveys of HIV/AIDS care and support, programme reports or other documents.

Monitoring and evaluation activities allow country health authorities and their partners to assess the extent to which programmes are being implemented and are achieving the intended objectives. Despite similarities, monitoring and evaluation differ in the extent to which findings at each level of service delivery can be attributed to a specific intervention or programme.

Monitoring aggregates information across sites and time and optimally serves as a tool to highlight for programme managers which programme components may need to be strengthened or modified to reach specific goals. It frequently counts the number of people receiving programme services. Monitoring data record programme input, processes and output.

Evaluation assesses the worth or value of a programme or collaboration between multiple programmes over time through more detailed analysis of their outcomes and, when possible, their impact on the target population. Evaluation can potentially link observed outcomes and impacts and the programme process. This is especially true when multiple agencies and programmes are working together and measuring the impact of efforts by individual partners is difficult; in these cases, impact measures may be inferred based on combined programme input, processes and output.

Tracking trends over time through routine monitoring and evaluation efforts will help programme managers and decision makers in assessing how successful programmes are in meeting goals. Most indicators are not designed to explain why a situation has or has not changed but to simply measure trends over time. A plan for collecting and analysing data should therefore be developed and focus on linking indicators that are collected at the various levels of the health care system.

Table 1 demonstrates how monitoring and evaluation are linked and provides examples of measures that can be collected at each level of effort.

Table 1

Monitoring and evaluation pipeline for HIVAIDS Care and Support

MONITORING "Process Evaluation"			*EVALUATION* "Effectiveness Evaluation"	
Inputs	*Process*	*Outputs*	*Outcome*	*Impact*
-Funds -Supplies/drugs -Equipment	-Training -HIV Testing -Treatment services HAART	-Trained staff -Clients receiving VCT; care; referred	-Improved provider attitudes -Improved community attitudes towards	-HIV-related morbidity -Mortality rate/life expectancy
-Policies, guidelines & procedures		-Clients receiving PLHA -receiving HBC -receiving PMTCT prescription	-Decreased discrimination -Restored productivity -Appropriate care delivery; referral; -Enhanced quality of life	

Input comprises the financial, material and human resources invested in care and support programmes and services. The process includes the types of activities a programme will deliver, such as training, HIV tests or drugs for treatment. Output refers to the deliverables from programme processes. such as the number of people served.

Outcome means the intermediate effects of programme efforts that are in accordance with programme objectives. For care and support, this may refer to changes in the capacity of the health system to deliver care, such as facilities with comprehensive care and support programmes necessary to care for people with HIV/AIDS, services complying with minimum standards, the quality of life of people served by programmes or the stigma-related attitudes of health care providers. Some of these measures in this example could appear at different levels depending on the specific programme objectives. The impact of care and support refers ultimately to physical and mental health - the morbidity and mortality rates of people living with HIV/AIDS, life expectancy and community productivity.

Conceptual Framework for Monitoring and Evaluation

A conceptual framework illustrates a model for monitoring and evaluating HIV/AIDS care and support activities. The model groups these indicators into strategic areas: developing and implementing policy; the capacity of health facilities, including human resources and access to antiretroviral drugs; the capacity of home- and community-based care; and the capacity to monitor and evaluate care and support.

The conceptual model also places each of these strategic areas at different levels, from global to national to programme. At the global level, the input of resources from international and multilateral agencies into the various strategic areas is measured. At the national level, this global input is synthesised for implementation in countries by national AIDS control programmes and other national administrative bodies. The programme level is where implementation takes place, ultimately affecting the burden of HIV/AIDS in a country. Methods for measurement are shown alongside each level.

National Capacity for Monitoring and Evaluation

Any discussion of the content of systems for monitoring and evaluating HIV/AIDS care and support must address national and international resources and the related systems for supporting these efforts. Indicators should be made as simple

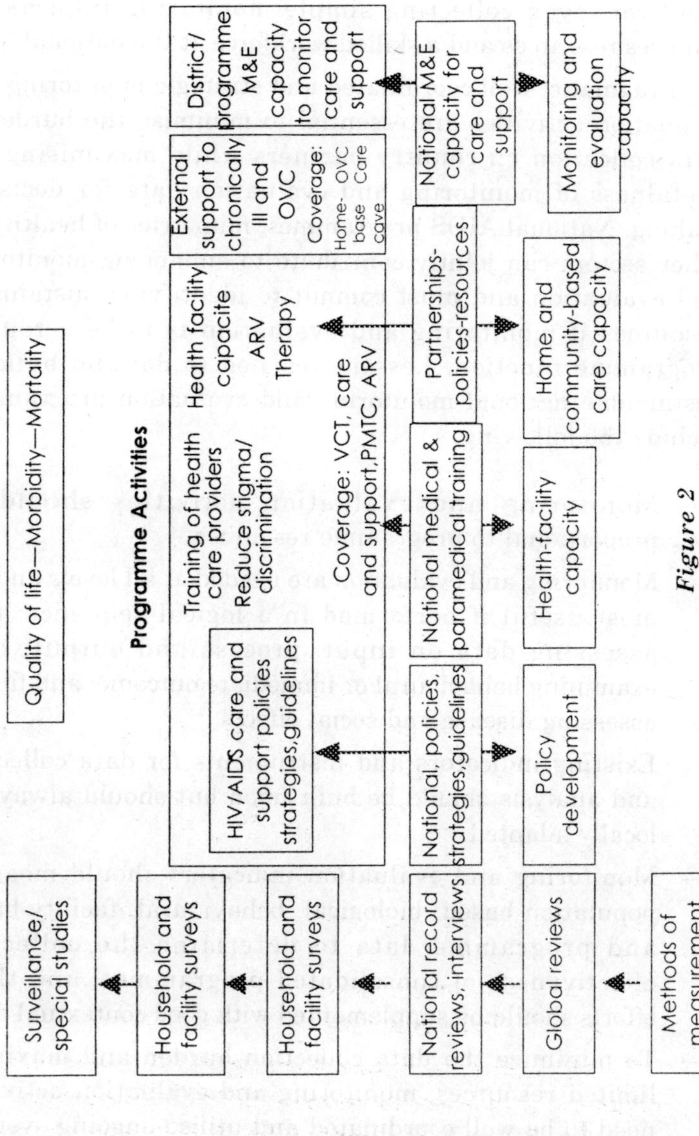

Figure 2

Conceptual Framework for Monitoring and Evaluation

and as complementary as possible to direct the most resources to achieving the ultimate objectives of these programmes. However, even collecting simple monitoring information requires resources and a skilled workforce at the national level.

Pragmatic, well coordinated and strategic monitoring and evaluation activities are essential to minimise the burden of data collection on country partners while maximising the usefulness of monitoring and evaluation data for decision-making. National AIDS programmes, ministries of health and other sectors can jointly contribute to enhancing monitoring and evaluation and must commit to identifying sustainable resources if monitoring and evaluation is to be a routine programme function. Lessons learned to date on building sustainable national monitoring and evaluation programmes include the following.

— Monitoring and evaluation activities should be proportional to programme resources.
— Monitoring and evaluation are needed at all levels and are most useful if performed in a logical sequence: first assessing data on input, process and output; then examining behavioural or immediate outcome; and finally assessing disease and social effects.
— Existing indicators and instruments for data collection and analysis should be built upon but should always be locally adapted.
— Monitoring and evaluation indicators should measure population-based, biological, behavioural, facility-based and programme data to determine the collective effectiveness of consolidated programmes, and these efforts should be supplemented with good contextual data.
— To minimise the data collection burden and maximise limited resources, monitoring and evaluation activities need to be well coordinated and utilise ongoing systems that collect and analyse data.

— To increase the utilisation of evaluation results, the design, planning, analysis and reporting of monitoring and evaluation should actively involve key stakeholders, such as district and national programme managers, policy-makers, community members and programme participants.

Maximising resources for developing and implementing a high-quality monitoring and evaluation framework, thus avoiding unnecessary duplication of efforts, requires that international partners work together. Bilateral donors, UNAIDS, WHO, the Global Fund for AIDS, Tuberculosis and Malaria, the World Bank and all their partners and cooperating agencies must work together to develop and evolve care and support indicators, standards and methods of monitoring and evaluation.

Indicators for Monitoring and Evaluation

The UNAIDS report, *Monitoring the Declaration of Commitment on HIV/AIDS: guidelines on construction of core indicators* provides a standardised set of indicators that can be used to monitor national programme goals. The list of indicators given in table 1 intentionally selected from significantly longer lists of potential indicators. The indicators presented here represent only key selected programme outputs and outcomes.

The indicators listed in Table 1 do not adequately measure quality, such as the quality of care, counselling or training. For example, the availability of trained staff is measured, but the indicator does not measure the quality of their training. The indicators included measure the basic external support received by chronically ill people and by affected orphans and vulnerable children, specifying a standard for receiving health, psychological and social services within a certain timeframe, but the quality of these services is not covered. In addition, the proposed indicators do not include feedback from people living with HIV/AIDS such as client interviews. To better understand

Table 2. List of Indicators

	Core indicators	*Recommended method*	*Frequency*
CS1	Percentage of the general population aged 15–49 years receiving HIV test results and post-test counselling in the past 12 months	Recommended method	Frequency
CS2	Percentage of districts with at least one health facility providing antiretroviral combination therapy	Programme reports	Annual
CS3	Percentage of people with advanced HIV infection receiving anti-retroviral combination therapy	Programme reports	Annual
CS4	Existence of comprehensive HIV/AIDS care and support policies, strategies and guidelines	Programme reports and modelling	Every 2 years
CS5	Percentage of facilities that provide comprehensive care referrals for HIV/AIDS care and support services (when these services are not available on site)	Interviews and record review	Every 2 years
CS6	Percentage of health facilities that have the capacity and conditionsto provide basic HIV counselling and testing and to manage HIV/AIDS clinical services a) A system for testing and providing results for HIV infection b) Systems and qualified staff for pre- and post-test counselling c) Specific health services relevant to HIV/AIDS, including resources and supplies for providing these services d) Elements for preventing nosocomial infections e) Trained staff and resources providing basic interventions for prevention and treatment for people living with HIV/AIDS	Health facility survey	Every 2–4 years
CS7	Percentage of health facilities that have the capacity and conditions to provide advanced HIV/AIDS clinical and psychosocial support services, including providing and monitoring antiretroviral combination therapy	Health facility survey	Every 2–4 years

(Contd...)

(Contd...)

	a) Systems and items to support the management of opportunistic infections and the provision of palliative care (symptomatic treatment) for the advanced care of people living with HIV/AIDS; b) Systems and items to support advanced services for the care of people living with HIV/AIDS c) Systems and items to support antiretroviral combination therapy d) Conditions to provide advanced inpatient care for people living with HIV/AIDS e) Conditions to support home care services f) Postexposure prophylaxis		
CS8	Percentage of designated laboratories with the capacity to monitor antiretroviral combination therapy according to national and international guidelines	Health facility survey or special laboratory study	To be determined
CS9	Percentage of adults aged 18–59 years who have been chronically ill for 3 or more months in the past 12 months whose households received, free of user charges, basic external support in caring for chronically ill adults, including health, psychological or emotional and other social and material support	Household survey	Every 2–4 years
CS10	Percentage of orphans and vulnerable children whose households received, free of user charges, basic external support in caring for the child	Household survey	Every 2–4 years
Additional indicators		*Method*	*Frequency*
CS-A1	Existence of national monitoring and evaluation capacity for HIV/AIDS care and support programmes	Interview or record reviews	Every 2 years
CS-A2	Percentage of health facilities with record-keeping systems for monitoring HIV/AIDS care and support	Health facility survey	Every 2–4 years

the content and quality of care for people living with HIV/AIDS, the indicators need to be complemented by additional questions related to the quality of care and support services and by qualitative methods such as focus groups, community advisory boards, client exit interviews, observation, mystery client or a combination of these.

During any pilot testing, the facility survey needs to consider the health system structure and to translate and adapt the instruments as necessary. For the household survey, special populations may need to be addressed in different ways. For high-prevalence countries, a nationally representative sample survey is appropriate, whereas for lower-prevalence countries or those with concentrated epidemics in select populations, implementing the survey methods may assess only the target population based on programmatic goals and objectives.

Sampling frames for the national level indicators rely on nationally representative samples of health facilities or households. The indicators presented above were field-tested in public and nongovernmental organisation programmes and facilities. Since private clinics may be providing critical services in many settings, such as anti-retroviral combination therapy, these need to be evaluated. Such services can be examined through special studies or can be included in the sampling frame by using oversampling techniques.

It was also decided for these indicators that only health facilities in the classic sense would be included in the sampling frame, thereby excluding institutions from health facility surveys such as groups of people living with HIV/AIDS or community based organisations that may be providing clinical services such as preventive therapy. However, because these types of organisations play an important role in providing care and support, programme managers may wish to adapt the methods to include such groups. This is especially true in settings in which these groups and the private sector in general play an important part in providing care and support services.

Although the indicators for care and support for orphans and vulnerable children and chronically ill people specify services free of user charges, this is not a requirement for the facility indicators. Critical issues such as the impact of human rights, stigma and discrimination and the access to care and treatment of special at risk populations should be further studied and addressed. In the facility survey, the highly diverse nature of clinics from country to country creates such structural challenges as the departments under which health workers will be sampled and the best way of assessing testing and counselling, clinical care services and appropriate referral when these services are administered in multiple sites or satellite sites within a health facility network.

Operations Research

Operations research is a rigorous kind of evaluation that can be used to improve a range of services along the full continuum of care for people living with HIV/AIDS and their families. It is most often used to compare programme approaches when there is no consensus about the best way to respond to a given programmatic problem. The main objective of operations research is to provide managers, administrators and policy-makers with the information they need to develop, improve or scale up programmes.

HIV/AIDS operations research focuses on the day-to-day activities or operations of HIV/AIDS prevention, care and support programmes. Specifically, it focuses on the aspects of programmes that are under the control of programme managers or policymakers, such as approaches to training and service delivery; the location, integration and distribution of services; or selecting health communication messages and materials needed to meet programme objectives.

Operations research can be thought of as a practical, systematic process for identifying and solving programme-related problems. This process has five key steps:

- — identifying and diagnosing a problem
- — selecting a programme strategy
- — testing and evaluating strategies
- — disseminating information
- — utilising information and scaling up.

The evolving areas of care and support, especially the increasing availability of treatment, require indepth studies on models of care to develop and implement the optimal delivery of services. Examples of specific areas of care and support that may require further indepth studies to enhance a comprehensive monitoring and evaluation framework include studies of anti-retroviral combination therapy and adherence, the quality of care, training of health care providers and the evolution of programmes and methods for monitoring stigma and discrimination within the health care system.

The strongest operations research studies strive to prove causality. That is, they are designed to prove that a given intervention brings about change and that this change would not have occurred in the absence of the intervention. Establishing this relationship requires designing a study in a manner that minimises potential confounding and bias while also providing results that are statistically significant.

Each of the following features helps in ensuring that a study meets these demands:

- — control or comparison groups;
- — baseline data collection;
- — multiple observations over time;
- — multiple sites;
- — multiple types of data collection;
- — research by an "objective" or outside party not affiliated with the programme;
- — multivariate data analysis; and

— emphasis on outcome indicators instead of process indicators.

MODELLING HIV/AIDS/STDs

Models for the spread of HIV vary in sophistication from straightforward curve fits to extremely complex process models reproducing the dynamics of multiple modes of transmission, requiring extensive behavioral, epidemiological, and demographic inputs. Both types of models have been applied by a number of different groups.

A strong demand has been seen for the output of these modelling efforts. This demand is driven by national AIDS programs and AIDS organisations, which wish to use them to advocate for expanded responses and to anticipate the magnitude of the tasks ahead of them, and by policy makers who want to understand the longer term implications of the epidemic for their own work.

The value of models comes not only from providing people with concrete estimates of HIV infections and deaths for advocacy and planning purposes, but because they force people to closely examine and try to coherently interpret available epidemiological and behavioral data.

In Asia-Pacific, epimodel, a simple cure fitting model, has been applied extensively. For the most part modelling efforts using process models have been concentrated in Thailand, with some additional work done in Indonesia and Papua New Guinea. All of this work currently exists as "gray literature," and not in published journals: The earliest and most extensive modelling efforts in the Asian region have looked at Thailand, perhaps encouraged by the ready availability of both epidemiological and behavioral data since 1990. Thailand also offers the best opportunity to check the validity of models, since eight years of epidemiological trend data along with numerous behavioural studies are available. A number of groups have examined the Thai epidemic.

The Thai experience is one of relatively abundant data, and an epidemiologically interesting and relatively complex (and in some respects an atypical) epidemic. Consequently, considerable modelling attention has been paid to the Thai case over the past decade.

Strong collaboration can help to ensure maximum use of available empirical data, while enhancing the chances for the results of modelling to be adopted by consensus and used in policy decisions and program planning.

But even in the same country using the same sources, considerable variation exists in the translation of epidemiological data into estimated current or cumulative prevalence figures. Further study is needed of how best to convert sentinel data sets to estimates of general population prevalence.

Trends in behavioural data are not easy to incorporate into existing models. The Thai situation in the 1990s has been a very dynamic one, which requires the ability to input behavioural parameters such as condom use and risk behavior over time if the epidemiological trends are to be reproduced.

Despite the complexity of some of the models, they have had limited success in fitting actual trends in the data, raising concerns about whether assumptions in the models correctly describe the complexity of the Thai situation.

Perhaps due to strong collaboration, examined even in hindsight, none of the above efforts produced results that were truly outlandish, although a number of such projections were to be found in the popular press. The higher results of the earliest efforts in part show the fact that much of the Thai behavior change had not yet been reflected in the data available.

Thailand has benefited substantially from these modelling efforts. Programmes and policies have been justified by the results of these models, and the Thai AIDS prevention effort has become stronger as a consequence. But the Thai experience also highlights the complexities of modelling AIDS epidemics and the potential pitfalls along the way. Other countries, perhaps with less empirical data and fewer resources devoted to modelling, have had differential success both in developing plausible models of the local epidemic as well as in incorporating these results into their prevention efforts

There is a need to improve policymakers understanding of uses and limitations of HIV/AIDS models. However, before that can be done, modellers themselves need to reach a consensus on the uses and limitations of the models that are in use in the developing countries. One approach to capacity building for modelling is to establish national technical working groups to assemble the relevant data and supervise the HIV estimation and projection process. These working groups can be linked through the Internet and convened through regional meetings.

Current modelling approaches perform best when an epidemic is in progress; tools for estimating levels and trends of HIV in the absence of an epidemic are not yet well developed. Alternative models need to be developed that include a few key variables and can describe the potential for an epidemic where HIV is still low. There is still a need in Asia for more capacity building in HIV and behavioural surveillance in order to collect the data that would be required by these models. Multi-country studies, with standardised methodology for collecting HIV/STD and behavioural data, should be applied along the lines of the current UNAIDS project in several countries in Africa. Application of complex process models to produce projections should be limited to countries in which at least three or four years of reliable epidemiological and behavioural trend data are available.

REFERENCES

d'Adesky, A., "Poor Countries Need Faster, Cheaper, Better HIV Monitoring", *The amfAR Treatment Insider*; 3(1): 1-5, 2002.

Fisher, A.A,, Foreit, J.R., *Designing HIV/AIDS Intervention Sudies: An Operations Research Handbook,* New York, Population Council, 2002.

UNAIDS, *National AIDS programmes: a guide to monitoring and evaluation,* Geneva, 2000.

______________, *Monitoring the Declaration of Commitment on HIV/AIDS: guidelines on construction of core indicators,* Geneva, 2002.

______________, *Monitoring and evaluation modules,* Geneva, 2002

United States Agency for International Development, *Expanded response guide to core indicators for monitoring and reporting on HIV/AIDS programmes,* Washington, DC, 2002.

WHO, *National AIDS programmes: A Guide to Monitoring and Evaluating HIV/AIDS Care and Support,* 2004.

Bibliography

Academy for Educational Development, *Fundamentals of HIV Prevention Counselling: Participants Manual*, 1998.

Aggleton, P. and I. Warwick, 1999, *Household and Community Responses to HIV and AIDS in Developing Countries: Findings from Multi-site Studies*, Geneva, UNAIDS.

Altman, D., *Power and Community: Organisational and Cultural Responses to AIDS*, London: Taylor and Francis, 1994.

Barnett E., De Koning K. and Francis V., "Health and HIV/AIDS Education in primary and secondary schools in Africa and Asia", *Education Research*, London, Department for International Development, 1995.

Barnett T. and Whiteside A., *AIDS in the Twenty–First Century*, Chippenham and Eastbourne, Antony Rowe Ltd., 2002.

Bharat, S. and P. Aggleton, "Facing the challenge: Household responses to AIDS in India," *AIDS Care* 11:33-46, 1999.

Blendon, R.J. and K. Donelan. 1988. "Discrimination against people with AIDS," *American Journal of Public Health* 319:1022-1026.

Bourdieu, P. and J-C. Passeron. 1977. *Reproduction in Education, Society and Culture*, London: Sage.

Bundy D., *Education and HIV/AIDS: A Window of Hope*, Washington DC, The World Bank, 2002.

Castells, M., *The Network Society*, Oxford: Blackwell Publishers, Inc., 1996.

Coombe, C., , Kelly M., "Education as a vehicle for combating HIV/AIDS", *UNESCO Prospects*; 31(3): 435–445), 2001.

Corbett, E.L., Watt, C.J., Walker, N., etal.. "The growing burden of tuberculosis: global trends and interactions with the HIV epidemic", *Archives of Internal Medicine*, 163:100-921, 2003.

Counselling for HIV/AIDS: a key to caring. For policy-makers, planners and implementors of counselling activities. Geneva: WHO, 1995.

d'Adesky, A., "Poor Countries Need Faster, Cheaper, Better HIV Monitoring", *The amfAR Treatment Insider*; 3(1): 1-5, 2002.

De Cock K.M., Fowler M.G., Mercier E, *et al*, "Prevention of mother-to-child HIV transmission in resource-poor countries–Translating research into pol policy and practice", *JAMA*, 2000; 283: 1175-82.

Dhaliwal, Mandeep, etal, *Scaling up HIV Testing and Counselling Services a toolkit for programme managers*, International HIV/AIDS Alliance, 2003.

Dunn D.T., Newell M.L., Ades A.E., *et al*, "Risk of human immunodeficiency virus type 1 transmission through breastfeeding", *Lancet*, 1992, 340:585-8.

Eastwood, A., and A. Maynard. 1988. Treating AIDS Patients: Is it Ethical to be Efficient" Paper presented at the First International Conference on the Global Impact of AIDS. London, March.

Egal F, Valstar A., *HIV/AIDS and nutrition: helping families and communities to cope*, Rome: Food and Agriculture Organisation, 2000.

EngenderHealth, *STI/HIV Prevention – Quick Reference Cards for Health Care Providers – What Every Client Should Know*, New York,2001.

EngenderHealth, *STI/HIV Prevention – Quick Reference Cards for Health Care Providers – What Every Client Should Know*, New York, 2001.

Fisher, A.A,, Foreit, J.R., *Designing HIV/AIDS Intervention Sudies: An Operations Research Handbook*, New York, Population Council, 2002.

From Principle to Practice: Greater Involvement of People Living with or Affected by HIV/AIDS (GIPA)", September 1999.

Gagnon, J.H. and W. Simon, *Sexual Conduct*. Chicago: Aldine, 1973.

Gilmore, N. and M.A. Somerville, "Stigmatisation, scapegoating and discrimination in sexually transmitted diseases, overcoming 'them' and 'us'," *Social Science and Medicine*, 39:1339-1358, 1994.

Global Programme on AIDS, "Consensus statement from the WHO/UNICEF consultation on HIV transmission and breastfeeding", *Weekly Epidemiological Record*, 1992, 67:177–179.

Gordon, G. and Gordon, P., *Counselling and Sexuality: A Video Based Training Resource*, IPPF, London, 1992.

Gostin, L.O. and Z. Lazzarini, *Human Rights and Public Health in the AIDS Pandemic*, New York: Oxford University Press, 1997.

Government of India, *National AIDS Contol Programme, HIV Testing Policy*, 1995.

ILO, *Action Against HIV/AIDS A Draft Framework for Global and Regional initiatives*, International Labour Organisation. Geneva, November 1999.

Increasing Access to HIV Testing and Counselling, WHO, 2002.

Institute of Medicine, National Academy of Sciences, *Mobilising Against AIDS*, Cambridge, Mass.: Harvard University Press, 1986.

Interim TB-HIV Guidelines, WHO, 2003.

Joint United Nations Programme on HIV/AIDS, *Counselling and HIV/AIDS: UNAIDS Technical Update*, November, 1997 .

Kegeles, S.M. etal., "Perceptions of AIDS, the continuing saga of AIDS-related stigma," *AIDS* 3(suppl.1):S253-S258, 1989.

Kelly M., *Planning for Education in the context of HIV/AIDS*, Paris, IIEP, UNESCO, 2000.

Kirp, D.L. and R. Bayer (ed.), 1992, *AIDS in the Industrialised Democracies*, New Brunswick, NJ: Rutgers University Press.

Leroy V., Newell M.L., Dabis F., *et al.*, "International multicentre pooled analysis of late postnatal mother-to-child transmission of HIV-1 infection", *Lancet*, 1998, 352:597-600.

Malcolm, A. et al., "HIV and AIDS-related stigmatisation and discrimination: its form and contexts." *Critical Public Health* 8(4):347-370, 1998.

Mann, J., D.J.M. Tarantola, and T.W. Netter (ed.), *AIDS in the World*, Boston, MA: Harvard University Press, 1992.

Mujeeb, S. 1999. "Human right violations of PLWA/HIV by their family members," posting to *SEA-AIDS*, Tue, 06 Jul 1999.

Ndondo, Noziqhu. T., "Preventing mother-to-child transmission of HIV. A training manual for healthcare providers". *Reproductive Health Alliance*, London, 2001.

Nduati R., Richardson B.A., John G., *et al*, "Effect of breastfeeding on mortality among HIV-1 infected women: a randomised trial", *Lancet*, 2001, 357:1651-5.

Opening the HIV/AIDS epidemic – Guidance of encouraging beneficial disclosure, ethical partner counselling &appropriate use of HIV case reporting, UNAIDS, 2001.

Opening the HIV/AIDS epidemic – Guidance of encouraging beneficial disclosure, ethical partner counselling &appropriate use of HIV case reporting. UNAIDS, 2001.

Parker, R.,"Administering the epidemic: HIV/AIDS policy, models of development and international health in the late-twentieth century," in *Globalisation, Health and Identity: The Fallacy of the Level Playing Field*, ed. L.M. Whiteford and L. Manderson. Boulder, CO: Lynne Rienner Publishing, pp. 39-55, 2000.

Pelletier, D.L., Frongillo Jr. E.A., Habicht J.P.," Epidemiologic evidence for a potentiating effect of malnutrition on child mortality", *Am J Public Health*, 1993, 83:1130-33.

Programme guidance on Counselling for STI/HIV prevention in sexual and reprodu ctive health settings, International Planned Parenthood Federation (IPPF), 2002.

Robert Holloway, "Lack of Awareness Hurts AIDS Prevention in Japan." *The Daily Yomiuri*, August 11, 1990.

Ronald Bayer, *Private Acts, Social Consequences: AIDS and the Politics of Public Health*, New Brunswick, M. J.: Rutgers University Press, 1991.

Sittitrai W., *Reproductive health and HIV/AIDS. Myanmar training manual: a community-based approach for youth and women*. Yangon, UNICEF, 1995.

Source book for HIV/AIDS counselling training. Geneva: WHO, 1994.

South African AIDS Training (SAT) Programme, *Basic counselling guidelines in HIV and AIDS*, July, 2001.

______________, *Counselling Guidelines on Child Sexual Abuse*. 2001.

______________, *Counselling Guidelines on Disclosure of HIV Status*. 2001.

______________, *Counselling Guidelines on Domestic Violence*, April. 2001.

South African AIDS Training (SAT) Programme. *Counselling Guidlines on Survival Skills for People Living with HIV*. 2001.

Sweat, M. and J. Dennison, "Reducing HIV incidence in developing countries with structural and environmental interventions." *AIDS* 9(suppl. A): S225-257, 1995.

Tarantola, and T.W. Netter. Boston, MA: Harvard University Press. UNAIDS, *HIV and AIDS-related stigmatisation, discrimination and denial: forms, contexts and determinants*, research studies from Uganda and India (prepared for UNAIDS by Peter Aggleton), Geneva, UNAIDS, 2000.

The Bangkok Collaborative Perinatal HIV Transmission Study Group, *Counselling Pregnant Women and New Mothers about HIV*. Produced by the HIV/AIDS Collaboration, Thailand, 1999.

The Right to Know: New Approaches in HIV Testing and Counselling. WHO, 2003.

Tirelli, U. etal, "HIV and discrimination", *British Medical Journal* 303:582, 1991.

UNAIDS policy on HIV testing and counselling, Geneva: UNAIDS, 1997.

UNAIDS, *Counselling and voluntary HIV testing for pregnant women in high prevalence countries: Guidance for service providers*, May, 1999.

UNAIDS, *National AIDS programmes: a guide to monitoring and evaluation*, Geneva, 2000.

UNAIDS, *Report on the global HIV/AIDS Epidemic*, 2002.

UNAIDS, Report on the global HIV/AIDS Epidemic, June 2000.

UNAIDS, UNICEF and WHO. *HIV and infant feeding. A policy statement developed collaboratively by UNAIDS, UNICEF and WHO*, Geneva, UNAIDS, 1997.

United States Agency for International Development, *Expanded response guide to core indicators for monitoring and reporting on HIV/AIDS programmes*, Washington, DC, 2002.

USAID, *USAID Concept Paper: Combating HIV/AIDS Stigma, Discrimination and Denial*, 2000.

VanDerslice J., Popkin B., Bris Briscoe J., "Drinking-water qual quality, sanitation, and breastfeed breastfeeding: Their interactive effects on infant health", *Bull WHO*, 1994: 72(4):589-601.

Voluntary Counselling and Testing (VCT), Paper for the UNAIDS expert panel on HIV testing in UN peacekeeping operations, 2001.

Voluntary Counselling and Testing (VCT): Program tools for implementing VCT, CDC, *Global AIDS Program*, April, 2003.

Walker N, Schwärtlander B., Bryce J., "Meeting international goals in child survival and HIV/ AIDS", *Lancet*, 2002. 360:284-9.

Welbourn, A., "Stepping Stones: A Training Package on HIV/AIDS, communication and relationship skills", *Strategies for Hope*, 1995.

Welbourn, A., "Stepping Stones: A Training Package on HIV/AIDS, communication and relationship skills", *Strategies for Hope*, 1995.

WHO, *National AIDS programmes: A Guide to Monitoring and Evaluating HIV/AIDS Care and Support*, 2004.

WHO, *New data on the prevention of mother-to-child transmission of HIV and the policy implications: conclusions and recommendations*, WHO technical consultation on the behalf of the UNFPA/UNICEF/WHO/UNAIDS Inter-Agency Task Team on Mother-to-Child Transmission of HIV, Geneva, 11-13 October 2000.WHO/RHR/01.28

World Bank, *Confronting AIDS: Public Priorities in a Global Epidemic*, New York: Oxford University Press, 1997.

World Health Organisation (WHO), *AIDS: Global Situation*, New Delhi, India: Southeast Asia Regional Office, 1992.

Index

Acquired Immune Deficiency Syndrome (AIDS) 1
ActionAid's approach 45
Ante-Natal Care (ANC) 188
Anti-retroviral combination therapy 274
Anti-Retro-Viral Drugs (ARVs) 25

Behavioural change 71
Behavioural Surveillance Surveys (BSS) 255
Biological resources 32

Civil society 82
Collectivism 12
Commodity management system 88
Communication skills 138
Community care programmes 114
Community empowerment 218
Community Mobilisation 85
Community-based
- Counselling 69
- Outreach 30
- Post-test 70
- Pre-test 70
- Programmes 229

Community-Based Organisations (CBOs) 39, 232
Complex regulatory environment 83
Comprehensive supportive services 260
Condom programmes 20
Conservation programmes 32
Contradictory information 54
Counselling organisations 225
Country co-ordinating mechanism (CCM) 130
Couple counselling 72
Criminal prosecution 216

Demographic and Health Survey (DHS) 41
Diagnostic testing 258
Discriminatory laws 83
Discriminatory practices 9
District-based delivery approaches 107
Drug Regulatory Authority (DRA) 85
Drug-using behaviour 156

Emotional exhaustion 74
Environmental interventions 19
Enzyme Immunoassays (EIAs) 93
Epidemiological reality 6
Epidemiological trend 275
Establish mechanisms 147

Formal education system 56
Focus Resources on Effective School Health (FRESH) 29

Gender equality, programmes 32
Gonorrhoea 142
Greater Involvement of People Living with or Affected by HIV/AIDS (GIPA) 19
Group counselling 139

Health Action International (HAI) 96
Health care systems 11
Health education theories 50
Heterosexual epidemic 6
Homophobia 11
Homosexuality 13
Human Immuno-deficiency Virus (HIV) 1
Human resources management 126
Human rights violations 230
Hypnotherapy 235

Immune system 239
Individualised voluntary counselling 106
Individualism 12
Information management systems 111
Information resources 30
Injecting drug users (IDU) 1
Intensive teacher training programme 65
Internally displaced persons (IDP) 116
International mobilisation 62
International policy frameworks 80
International programmes 264
Interpersonal interaction 76

Life skills approach 55
Low-risk behaviour 230

Medecins sans Frontieres (MSF) 96
Men who have sex with men (MSM) 1
Micronutrient supplements 197
Morally deplorable behaviour 48

National Drug (Medicines) Programme 93
Non-discriminatory practices 233
Non-governmental organisations (NGOs) 77, 229

Opt-out approaches 79
Organisation of Eastern Caribbean States (OECS) 98

Parent-teacher associations 47
Partner counselling programme 143
Passive surveillance system 250
Peace-keeping forces 3
People living with HIV/AIDS (PLHA) 9
Physical education (PE) 55
Polygamy 24
Post-exposure prophylaxis (PEP) 84
Postnatal transmission 198
Poverty Reduction Strategy Papers 33
Pre-marital counselling 171
Premarital counselling. 72
Pre-qualification scheme 92, 100
Prevention and care programmes 228
Prevention mother-to-child HIV transmission (PMTC 84
Prevention services 2

Preventive therapy 272
Programme resources 268
Promiscuity 13
Psychological dimensions 17
Psychological stress reduction 72
Public health approach 79
Public information campaigns 231

Qualitative research 62
Quality assurance system 117
Quality improvement processes 111

Racism 11
Referral system 263
Referral Systems 78
Reflexology 235
Regulatory systems 99
Reproductive Tract Infection (RTI) 154
Resource mobilisation 81
Rights-based approach 29
Risk behavioral questions 256

Safe sexual behaviour 59
Self-help groups 221
Sero-conversion 198
Service delivery approach 110
Sex-related Stigma 6
Sexual harassment 180
Sexuality 148
Sexually Transmitted Diseases (STDs) 4
Sexually Transmitted Infections (STIs) 24
Social isolation 5
Social security systems 2
Socio-behavioral investigations 256
Spiritual support 133
Stigma and discrimination (S&D) 6
Stigma of 6 Class-related 7 Fear-related 8
Stress management 225
Supply management cycle 103,104
Surveillance systems, design of 253
Survival skills 220
Syphilis 142

Therto-child transmission services 27
Total Health Programme 56
Traditional medicinal plants 30

United Nations General Assembly Special Session (UNGASS) 195
Universal HIV screening programmes 252
Universal Precautions (UP) 84
Voluntary Counselling and Testing (VCT) 188

Work-related policies 35
World Health Organisation (WHO) 29, 250

Zinc, vitamins A, C, and E and selenium (ZACES) 238